MULTI-INSTITUTIONAL HOSPITAL SYSTEMS

Howard S. Zuckerman, Ph.D.
Principal Author
Lewis E. Weeks, Ph.D.
Editor

This publication and the projects on which it is based were supported by grants from the W. K. Kellogg Foundation.

Hospital Research and Educational Trust
Chicago, Illinois

Library of Congress Cataloging in Publication Data

Zuckerman, Howard S   1939-
    Multi-institutional hospital systems.

    "HRET catalog number: 9160."
    1. Multihospital systems. 2. Multihospital
systems—United States—Case studies. I. Weeks,
Lewis E. II. Title. [DNLM: 1. Hospital adminis-
tration—United States. 2. Hospital shared services.
WX150.3 Z94m]
RA971.Z82   658'.91'36211   79-23586
ISBN 0-87914-054-2

©1979 by the
Hospital Research and Educational Trust
840 North Lake Shore Drive
Chicago, Illinois 60611

All rights reserved
Printed in the U.S.A.

HRET T-497

Designed and printed by:
Visual Images Inc.
Des Plaines, Illinois

Foreword

Perhaps the most important changes in health care in the 1970s have been structural and organizational, not medical or technological. This publication highlights one of those changes as it describes the "state of the art" of the multihospital or multi-institutional system movement–the issues that have surfaced out of this restructuring, the literature available, and, most importantly, the very significant impact that the Kellogg Foundation has had upon this development by funding several successful demonstration projects.

As we look to the 1980s, it is apparent that the multihospital system and other multi-institutional arrangements have moved through a very important first phase. In the first phase, the managers of hospitals and other health care institutions have become more accustomed to the broadened responsibilities of a corporate kind of structure, more secure about interinstitutional relationships, and more willing to trade some institutional autonomy for new access to broader community health delivery programs. The concept has been put into place and the industry has accepted it.

Government has carefully monitored the changes that are taking place, and is becoming more supportive of multi-institutional arrangements. Indeed, if the multihospital system performance is good, it may well serve to protect the private sector from additional government encroachment.

As one observes the development of the next phase of this movement, one should expect some important new considerations. Competition between systems for future growth will be a major factor, particularly between the large voluntary and investor-owned systems. There will be increased need for corporate planning, data base development, (with particular emphasis on linkages of financial and clinical systems), and operations research for management. There will also be a growing need for assessment of system performance and documentation of the economic and political implications of the maturing system structures.

The 80s will also see a more distinct delineation of the various kinds of systems. Regional systems, affiliated chains of voluntary hospitals, along with investor-owned chains, and religious systems will each take on a somewhat different approach to the development and management of their systems. As that occurs, hospital associations will also have to rethink their role as coordinators of shared services.

We may also expect to see the multi-institutional corporation begin to seriously explore an important role in financing care. A strategy that may be increasingly pursued as a result of competition would be for the multi-institutional organization to accept an insurance risk for a certain population, either as an insurer or in cooperation with an insurer. Such an arrangement would add to the incentive to form affiliations with other providers in order to achieve economies, and enhance efforts at regionalization.

Whatever shape or structure these systems develop, they will have to look beyond the multihospital system to a broader comprehensive delivery system that encompasses all health delivery in the community. Health care leadership will have to recognize that to successfully meet the challenges of the future, even more new relationships must develop between existing organizations, and new organizations must develop with new perspectives on community health delivery.

Each of us recognizes the true value of the individual community hospital as the focal point for community health. However, a combination of factors–cost, organizational size, ability to develop a minimum mass of management and clinical specialists, social and political pressures within the small organization, and an inability to out maneuver other socioeconomic structures in the community–make it increasingly difficult for the individual institution or a small system to effectively influence community health delivery.

Besides the need for broader interinstitutional arrangements, these systems have to reach out to the academic medical centers and seek an integration of the care and manpower production elements of health.

Herein lies the potential for a comprehensive system that is manpower-self-sufficient, cost-effective, and one with the ability to integrate its care systems both vertically and horizontally.

The system we seek in the 1980s may well be a unified comprehensive health care delivery system with a core teaching hospital and multiple other hospitals and health care delivery mechanisms that:

1. Balances the health care needs both socioeconomically and geographically in the inner city, urban, suburban, and rural communities.

2. Develops a more rational system for achieving quantitative and qualitative balance in the production and assignment of health manpower.

3. Provides continuing education for health professionals that reduces the gap between advances in technology and application.

4. Attempts to achieve economies and diversity of experience by sharing clinical and institutional facilities.

5. Recognizes cost-effective management of the health care system is contingent upon multihospital systems, participation in the solution of the problems of manpower production and participation by academic medical centers in the solution of the problems of horizontal and vertical integration of care.

The systems of the future that achieve this integration should be able to achieve regionalization, a pooling of resources, and a sharing and concentration of power with the ability to test the parameters of government regulation never seen before in the health care industry.

Gail L. Warden
Chicago, Illinois
July 10, 1979

Preface

This book is concerned with the growth and development of multi-institutional systems, a phenomenon that is reconfiguring the structure of the hospital industry. This volume begins with a "state-of-the-art" paper, representing an attempt to outline some of the key issues relevant to these systems. The paper offers a typology of interorganizational arrangements, presents the "promise" of multihospital systems, and assesses the "performance" of the systems in light of their promise. Environmental and organizational barriers to achievement of the potential are considered and areas of further opportunity for system development are discussed. It should be noted that a good deal of the source material for this section was provided by the American Hospital Association Center for Multihospital Systems and Shared Services Organizations. The Center made available many of the papers presented at recent conferences on multihospital systems, and these papers proved invaluable in preparing this section of the book. The establishment of the Center is testimony to the recognition of the growing importance of multi-institutional arrangements. Particular thanks are due to Bob Toomey, Consulting Director of the Center, and to Scott Mason, Staff Specialist, for their assistance.

The second part of the book includes case descriptions of 10 selected multi-institutional systems. In each instance the W. K. Kellogg Foundation provided "seed money" for system growth and development. The descriptions seek to provide information on the background and purpose of each system, the organizational structure, operating processes, and, to the extent possible, resultant outcomes. Special thanks go to David P. Smith and Kathryn Walker, who joined me in the writing of these case descriptions. David and Kathryn, graduate students in the Program in Hospital Administration at the University of Michigan at the time of this writing, assumed substantial responsibility in the preparation of this section. We are certainly grateful to the many individuals within the 10 systems with whom we discussed our work for their cooperation and assistance in this effort.

The final section of the book includes three papers selected from recent conferences. These papers were chosen because of their important insights and perceptions regarding the multihospital movement. They offer commentary on a number of fundamental concerns about the growth and development of systems, including purposes, roles, opportunities, and constraints.

A special note of appreciation should be made to the W. K. Kellogg Foundation. The Foundation initiated this project, and through their interest and funding, made possible its completion. The Hospital Research and Educational Trust is also due my gratitude for their continuing support throughout this effort.

In addition, several other acknowledgements are in order. My thanks to my good friend and colleague, Bob Vraciu, for his thoughtful review of earlier drafts; to my Program Director, John Griffith, for providing me with the time and resources to work on this project; to my secretary, Ruth Calkins, and to Mary Ann Guenther, for typing the many revisions; to Lew Weeks for his advice and counsel and for his thorough editorial review; and to my family for their patience and tolerance over the last several months.

Howard S. Zuckerman, Ph.D.
Ann Arbor, Michigan
June 14, 1979

Contents

Forward   i

Preface   v

Part I Multi-Institutional Systems   1

Multi-Institutional Systems: Their Promise and Performance   3
Howard S. Zuckerman, Ph.D.

Part II Case Descriptions   53

Introduction   55

Billings Deaconess Hospital   57

Carolinas Hospital and Health Services, Inc.   67

Eastern Maine Medical Center   83

Fairview Community Hospitals, Inc.   91

Henry Ford Hospital   105

Health Central, Inc.   117

Nebraska Methodist Hospital   133

Presbyterian Hospital Center   143

Saginaw General Hospital   155

Virginia Mason Medical Center   167

Summary   179

Part III Selected Conference Papers   183

The Issues Facing Multihospital Systems   185
  Robert M. Sigmond

Generic Problems in the Development and
Operation of Multihospital Systems   199
  Edward J. Connors

Impact on and Opportunities for
Multihospital Systems and Shared
Service Organizations   207
  Donald C. Wegmiller

Part I

Multi-Institutional Systems: Their Promise and Performance

Multi-Institutional Systems: Their Promise and Performance

*Howard S. Zuckerman**

Introduction

> Centuries ago, in rural England, 'the commons' was a grazing field open to all individuals in a community. Each, addressing his own individual needs, placed further cattle upon it until the green grass died. 'The tragedy of the commons' was that no mechanisms existed for confronting each person with the inevitable fate that linked him to his fellows. All societies, this one in particular, had placed some value upon individualism and competition. This works so long as resources are relatively infinite compared with the demands placed upon them. Today resources are not infinite, and tasks are so complex that neither individuals nor single organizations can perform them altogether effectively. We are in an era of interdependence.[1]

This quotation aptly describes the environment of our times. Traditionally, hospitals have existed as freestanding, autonomous institutions, largely in control of their own destiny. In recent years, however, pressure has mounted to contain costs, to rationalize the delivery of care, to reduce unnecessary duplication of facilities and services, to increase the availability of and access to care, and to improve quality. While various legislative and regulatory schemes have been proposed or enacted as presumed remedies, what has been lacking is an examination of the

* Assistant Professor and Associate Director, Program and Bureau in Hospital Administration, The University of Michigan.

3

basic structure of the hospital industry. The growth and development of multi-institutional arrangements represents an attempt, through organizational integration and consolidation, to restructure the industry from within in order to effectively meet the challenges being faced. Increasingly, hospitals are recognizing the need to work together, joining resources and skills. The signals are clear–increased regulation, rising consumer expectations, limited dollars, concern over costs–that we are witnessing the decline of autonomous, individual institutions and the growth of new collaborative forms of organization.[2,3,4,5,6]

Although multi-institutional arrangements are recent phenomena in terms of growth, the idea is not a new one. Some 50 years ago, the Committee on the Costs of Medical Care advocated such arrangements,[7] and the Hill-Burton legislation in 1946 was also supportive of this notion. In 1962, McNerney and Riedel suggested interorganizational coordination in rural areas through regionalization.[8] The American Hospital Association, in its 1965 Statement on Optimum Health Services, indicated the need for "coordinated community and regional systems of facilities and services."[9] The 1968 Report of the Secretary's Commission on Hospital Effectiveness (Barr Report) noted the desirability of "combinations of hospitals as well as inter-hospital cooperation and coordination."[10] Both the Regional Medical Programs and the Comprehensive Health Planning Act of the mid-1960s clearly intended regionalization, cooperation, and integration of facilities and resources. More recently, the Health Resources Planning and Development Act of 1974 (P. L. 93-641) provides specific encouragement for interorganizational arrangements. In listing 10 national priorities to be used in health planning efforts, the Congress explicitly refers to such arrangements several times, urging:

- The development of multi-institutional systems for coordination or consolidation of institutional health services (including obstetric, pediatric, emergency medical, intensive and coronary care, and radiation therapy services).
- The development of medical group practices (especially those whose services are appropriately coordinated or integrated with institutional health services), health maintenance organizations, and other organized systems for the provision of health care.
- The development of health service institutions of the capacity to provide various levels of care (including intensive care, acute general care, and extended care) on a geographically integrated basis.
- The development of multi-institutional arrangements for the sharing of support services necessary to all health service institutions.[11]

Recent data, presented in Table 1, provides evidence of the magnitude of the development of interorganizational arrangements. Reporting on short-term community hospitals, Brown and Lewis found that, in 1975, 24 percent of community hospitals and 32 percent of community hospital beds were part of multiple hospital systems.[12] The data indicate that the for-profit sector already is dominated by investor-owned systems and that there is extensive penetration of systems in the not-for-profit sector as well. Upward of 370 multiple hospital systems are said to be operating in the United States, and the degree of concentration within the industry appears to be growing.

TABLE 1

Community Hospitals and Beds in Multiple
Hospital Systems, by Type of Ownership - 1975

Type of Ownership	Total Hospitals	Hospital Systems	%	*Total Beds	*Hospital Systems	%
Nongovernmental, not-for-profit	3,355	940	28	649,000	210,000	32
Investor-owned, for-profit	755	309	40	70,000	37,000	51
State and local government	1,745	156	8	207,000	46,000	22
TOTAL	5,855	1,405	24	926,000	293,000	32

*rounded numbers

Source: Montague Brown and Howard L. Lewis. *Hospital Management Systems-Multi-Unit Organization and Delivery of Health Care,* Germantown, MD: Aspen Systems Corporation, 1976.

Organizational Typologies

Multiple institutional arrangments may be defined as any combination of individual facilities under a consolidated or cooperative structure which serves to form a larger entity. This is a broad definition, recognizing that these arrangements have evolved taking a variety of organizational forms. A number of efforts have been made to categorize and describe these various alternatives. Clark, for example, has suggested that systems might be characterized in terms of the degree of their physical or organizational integration.[13] Starkweather, in his formulation, includes geographic proximity of facilities and organizational patterns in a manner similar to Clark, but he adds five additional dimensions: (1) "legal bonds," which range from implied agreements to formal agreements which replace all prior legal entities; (2) "nature of combined services," ranging from support and administrative services only to direct patient care operations; (3) "stages and forms of production," ranging from affiliations between different organizations to transformations which lead to new forms of health care delivery; (4) "geography of population served," in contrast with geography of provider organizations; and (5) "organizational impact," which ranges from minimal changes in individual tasks or jobs to systemwide changes, unexpected impact, and unpredictable consequences.[14] Each of these seven dimensions may be viewed as a spectrum of arrangements among institutions, representing various types and degrees of interorganizational cooperation.

DeVries, in a recent effort, has developed a scheme by which to categorize multiple hospital arrangements.[15] Using corporate ownership, corporate management, and system influence on major policy decisions as the dimensions of interest, DeVries suggests seven types of organizational arrangements. Ranging across a continuum of increasing system control, the categories include formal affiliation, shared or cooperative services, consortia for planning or education, contract management, lease, corporate ownership but separate management, and complete ownership. Variations on these basic themes have been suggested by Mason[16] and by Reynolds and Stunden.[17] For purposes of reviewing the current status of interorganizational arrangements and to point to some recent developments, a formulation drawing primarily on DeVries and Starkweather will be used. Emphasis will be placed on ownership, degree of management centralization, extent of policy control, and geographic proximity of facilities. The types of arrangements to be included fall into two major categories–multiple ownership and single ownership. Within each of these categories, the predominant organizational forms will be discussed.

Multiple Ownership

Shared Services

The first category of interest is that of shared services or affiliations, representing the least pervasive types of arrangment between two or more organizations. Consolidation applies only to a specific program or service, which may be clinical or administrative in nature. Within the joint or shared venture, all participating parties are at risk.[18] Ownership of the participating institutions continues to be separate, management remains decentralized, and major policy control is retained by each separate

organization. Geographic proximity can vary in shared service or affiliation arrangements. That is, there are illustrations of services shared
among organizations in geographic proximity, for example shared laundry services, as well as services such as joint purchasing, which can be
shared by organizations that are geographically dispersed.

Sharing of services among institutions is widespread. A 1971 survey of
short-term community hospitals indicated that two-thirds of the
responding hospitals were involved in some form of sharing.[19,20] An extensive list of shared services was categorized into four groups: medical
facilities and care, manpower resources, administrative and other services, and continuing education/in-service training programs. Results indicated that the greatest concentration of sharing was in the area of administrative services and secondarily in medical facilities and care. While
blood banking, a medical service, was reported as the single most frequently shared service, eight of the next nine most common shared services were administrative in nature. Among the eight, purchasing of
various types of supplies was predominant.

Taylor, in 1975, found evidence of substantial sharing among hospitals
of all types, with the greatest degree of participation occurring in short-
term general community hospitals, particularly nongovernmental, not-
for-profit facilities.[21] Administrative services remained the most frequently shared, led by purchasing, electronic data processing,
educational training, laundry, insurance programs, credit and collection,
and management engineering. Most commonly shared clinical services
included blood banking, laboratory services, and diagnostic radiology.
The data indicate significant expansion of sharing since 1970, with the
rate of growth for administrative services exceeding that of clinical services.

Sharing of services has taken place within various types of arrangements. Among the alternatives are: *referred* services, in which one institution provides the services to other participating institutions; *purchased* or
joint contract services, where a group of institutions has cooperatively
negotiated one contract with one provider of a service or resource;
multisponsored services, in which the service is organized and operated on
a cooperative basis by the participating institutions, often through creation of a separate organization; and *regional* service, which is organized
and operated through a local, state, or regional association.[22]

A recent development is the emergence of shared activities across
multihospital systems. Such intersystem sharing is evidenced by the creation of Associated Hospital Systems (AHS), a group composed of 10
nonprofit multihospital systems with some 240 facilities and almost

29,000 beds.[23] Also of interest is the formation of the Voluntary Hospitals of America, Inc. (VHA), a for-profit cooperative which includes some 30 large hospitals and hospital systems.[24] Fitschen has argued that the for-profit mode will enable the cooperative to avoid certain restrictions on the scope of its activities and to allow for retention of profits.[25] In both AHS and VHA, shared purchasing represents an area of initial activity. Of special note is the move to expand such purchasing into the realm of capital equipment. Traditionally, joint purchasing has focused on low unit cost, high volume supplies. The move to joint capital purchasing suggests concern with low volume, high unit cost equipment. These two groups continue to explore common problems and seek to identify areas of potential for shared arrangements. Overall, shared services represents a growing form of interorganizational activity.

Consortia

The second type of arrangement is the consortium, a cooperative venture in which a group of institutions engage in joint planning, notably for clinical services. The institutions involved usually are geographically proximate, and their activities may result in a reallocation of clinical and medical services for a geographically definable population. Within a consortium, each hospital maintains its corporate ownership and identity, but a central coordinating body typically is established. Thus, consortia do influence major policy decisions for member hospitals but do not affect management control.

While the basic thrust is in joint planning, several consortia have been active in sharing both clinical and management services. Coordination and integration of medical staffs has also been a component of much of the consortia effort. While the membership of a consortium may include diverse types and different size institutions, a common theme is recognition of the equality and interdependency among the participating organizations.[26,27,28]

Management Contracts

A third category is the management contract, or full management without ownership. In this arrangement, the servicing organization assumes full responsibility for day-to-day management. Ownership and legal responsibility, however, are retained by the managed institution. The servicing agency does exert some influence on major policy decisions, and management contracts have been arranged between organizations both geographically proximate and geographically dispersed. Brown has argued that such an arrangement allows the servicing organization to grow and expand while the managed facility receives needed skills and expertise.[29,30]

In the not-for-profit sector, several recent surveys indicate that the management contract has been and will continue to be a rapidly growing approach to interorganizational arrangements.[31,32] Of particular note is the increasing use of management contract arrangements by small, rural hospitals, often faced with severe financial, service, and manpower problems.[33,34,35]

Within the investor-owned sector, management contracts have, for some time, been viewed as a desirable means of organizational growth.[36,37] Among many of the investor-owned systems, management contracts are expected to be a major area of expansion, although there will be continued activity in acquisition of existing hospitals or building of new hospitals.[38,39,40] It might be added that the investor-owned systems, while primarily servicing for-profit hospitals, have contracted to manage a number of nonprofit hospitals as well. While early contracts often involved hospitals which were in very serious difficulty, management companies are now showing increasing selectivity, looking for institutions which could be viable or are already doing reasonably well but which could still benefit from the arrangement.[41]

The recent growth and development of mangement contracts in both the nonprofit and for-profit sectors is summarized below in Table 2.

TABLE 2

Growth and Development of Management Contracts

| | 1977 | | 1978 | |
	Facilities	Beds	Facilities	Beds
Nonprofit	35	3,756	46	5,038
For-profit	240	25,810	290	34,195

Source: Donald E. L. Johnson. "87 multi-hospital systems grew 10%; predict 9% expansion in 1979." *Modern Healthcare,* 9:46, April 1979.

Leases

A lease arrangement is somewhat similar to a management contract in that it provides full management without ownership. However, a major distinction is that under a lease arrangement major policy decisions are made by a corporate board separate from the owners of the managed institution. In essence, the lease transfers possession of hospital property and equipment, for a specified number of years and for a specified rental, along with responsibility for the operation and maintenance of the hospital. The board of trustees of the leased hospital often continues to exist, albeit in an advisory capacity. Thus, control of both policy and management are assumed by the leasing organization. Lease arrangements do not appear to be constrained geographically in that there are examples both proximate and dispersed.[42,43]

Single Ownership

Decentralized

Within the single corporate ownership model, the first category is characterized by separate or decentralized governance and management. There is usually modest system influence on major policy decisions of the individual hospitals. The hospitals, often geographically dispersed, are typically full service institutions with their own community boards of trustees. Thus, while legal ownership is centralized and there may be a corporate level management staff, there remains a high degree of management and policy autonomy at the local level. Exemplifying this type of structure is the not-for-profit chain of a religious order, such as those owned and operated by Catholic orders. *SISTERS OF MERCY*

In recent years, concern for the continued viability of Catholic sponsorship has led to discussion of a number of possibilities for restructuring *1* these chains.[44,45] Among the alternatives proposed, one model would have Catholic hospitals either adding other Catholic hospitals to their systems under the same ownership or serving other Catholic hospitals *2* through shared services or management contracts. A second alternative would be to add, through acquisition, hospitals from different congregations, necessitating a change in corporate structure to reflect the new af- *3* filiation. Third, large Catholic hospitals might provide management con- *4* tract services to smaller, often rural, Catholic hospitals. A fourth possibility is a consortium among Catholic hospitals, located within *5* defined geographic and political boundaries. Yet another alternative suggested is the creation of an umbrella corporation or holding company, through which shared services and management support could be provided to participating institutions and which could serve as a base from which to assume management responsibility or ownership of other hospitals.[46] Thus, a broad and far reaching set of possibilities are under consideration as alternatives to the currently predominant model.

Centralized

The second type of single ownership is that within which governance and management are largely centralized. A variety of types of arrangements fall within this category, including satellites, holding companies, investor-owned chains, hospital authorities, and mergers. All of these are structured such that the central corporate offices control major policy decisions. Management control tends to be centralized, although there is some variation among the several arrangements. Among nonprofit systems there are instances of both geographic proximity and dispersion within this category.

An example of the centralized single corporate ownership type is the satellite or branch facility, which may be a hospital or ambulatory care center. The satellite, spun off by an existing hospital, is often located in a suburban area while the parent organization is located in an urban setting. There is a single board of trustees, a single medical staff, and the administrative staff is employed by the corporate organization. These satellite arrangements have served to respond to population shifts, thus expanding patient markets and referral networks.[47,48]

Also illustrative of this category is the hospital holding company, patterned after an approach common in the banking industry. There is typically a corporate board, with representation from member institutions, as well as local advisory boards. Corporate level staff specialists are available for management consultation. In some cases, a regional executive may oversee a group of member institutions.[49] The holding company approach is designed to centralize control of policy and capital allocation decisions at the corporate level, while retaining decentralization and local autonomy for operating responsibility.[50,51,52] The investor-owned chains often are structured along these lines, although the degree of decentralization for operating decisions varies across the corporations.[53]

Yet another example of centralized single ownership is the merger. Merger occurs where two or more previously independent organizations come together to form a new organization through either (a) pooling assets, with each organization losing its identity to form a separate, new corporation or (b) acquisition, with one organization dissolving and being absorbed by another.[54] By definition, all policy and management control is centralized within the newly formed organization. Merger often occurs among urban institutions in geographic proximity and with overlapping markets or service areas.

There are, then, a variety of arrangements by which multi-institutional systems have evolved. The systems vary in terms of ownership, policy and management control and centralization, and geographic dispersion. A review of the typologies proposed thus far indicates that they are probably not exhaustive nor are the categories mutually exclusive. Some of the organizational types discussed are in fact a mix of several categories. For instance, holding companies may have members included via mergers or satellites, and they also may be involved in sharing services and providing lease arrangements and management contracts. Rather than discrete organizational types, what we may be witnessing is a cumulative scale as one moves along an increasingly pervasive continuum of integration. Further, while a number of organizational arrangements have been described, certain of these represent identifiable *structures* but others may be more appropriately viewed as *processes* by which organizations coordinate or consolidate activities. The classifications developed to date offer a sound foundation to begin to understand the ways in which interorganizational arrangements have developed. It is equally clear, however, that there is yet work to be done in the formulation of organizational typologies.

The Promise of Multi-Institutional Systems

As multi-institutional systems have evolved, a number of potential benefits have been ascribed to them. Three types of benefits are described, categorized as economic, manpower, and organizational. Further, these benefits may be viewed at two levels. The first, the institutional level, refers to that set of advantages to be secured by the multi-institutional systems per se and/or by their individual members. The second, or community level, refers to the benefits presumed to accrue to the people served by these systems. The promise of multi-institutional systems may thus be framed in terms of benefits to providers and/or consumers. Such a formulation will enable us to evaluate the performance of multi-institutional arrangements in light of these anticipated benefits.

Economic Benefits

The first type of benefit revolves around the notion of economies of scale. At the institutional level, organizational consolidation should lead to improved utilization of resources, both capital and operating. Increased size should enable the system, through coordinated activities, to meet the same level of demand with less capacity than that required by separate facilities.[55] This advantage is particularly relevant for systems which are geographically proximate. Larger scale of operations also allows for specialization of personnel and equipment, increased productivity, and lower staffing requirements.[56,57]

Another potential economic benefit lies in the ability of systems to secure capital financing unavailable to freestanding institutions. The strength of systems provides improved access to capital markets, reduced costs of borrowing money and the sharing of financing fees. Systems are viewed as a lower credit risk since the financial risk of individual facilities is spread over a larger operating and financial base.[58,59,60]

Economies of scale are also expected from shared services activities such as joint purchasing, which allows large volume buying, lower unit costs, and greater discounts for the participating institutions.[61,62] Many of these economic benefits are applicable across the continuum of system configurations.

A number of the economic advantages cited at the institutional level may also accrue to the communities being served. For example, larger scale of operations may lead to reduced operating costs which, in turn, may result in lower prices to consumers.[63] Multi-institutional systems may also serve to rationalize the planning process. By coordinating development of programs and services, systems can move toward planning at the community or regional level rather than focusing solely on individual hospitals.[64] This rationalization of the planning process may be a means to avoid duplication of facilities and services, to improve the allocation of resources, and to reduce excess capacity.[65] At the community level, benefits of such rationalization have both economic and qualitative implications.

Manpower Benefits

For the second type of benefit, manpower, it has been argued that systems have advantages at the institutional level in terms of recruitment and retention of both clinical and administrative personnel. For clinicians, there is generally a broader range of services and programs, different levels of care, and access to specialized personnel and equipment. Availability of specialists allows for consultation, continuing education, expanded patient referral networks, and simplification of vacation and educational leaves.[66] A stronger and more integrated clinical organization has been said to lead to improved quality of care throughout the system, and coupled with a more complete data base, may lead to innovation in peer review processes.[67]

A strong management capability is seen as vital to coping with an increasingly complex environment. The capability of systems to attract and keep competent managers is considered a major attribute.[68] At the corporate level, the organization can use its greater management capacity to strengthen the system in total. At the individual institutional level, hospitals have access to specialized management talent and may be in a stronger position to recruit inhouse administrative personnel. Multi-institutional systems can provide improved professional opportunities and a stimulating managerial environment.[69] Systems often consist of different types and sizes of institutions in various geographic locations, offering managers career mobility while enabling them to remain within the system.[70] It has also been suggested that the availability of a sound management structure, along with financial stability, is an attractive feature in the recruitment and retention of physicians.[71]

The ability to recruit and retain clinical and administrative manpower can be advantageous not only to the institutions involved but to the community served as well. Systems can attract high quality clinical personnel, can offer greater technical expertise and specialization, and improve the distribution of health manpower.[72] Likewise, greater depth and expertise in management should provide for stronger, more viable organizations to serve the population. To the extent that such manpower availability serves to enhance quality of care, people being served by systems thereby benefit.

Organizational Benefits

The third area, organizational benefits, is also perceived to accrue from the development of multi-institutional arrangements. At the institutional level, these arrangements represent opportunities to expand service areas, increase market penetration, and open new patient referral networks, thus providing for organizational growth.[73] For institutions in underserved areas, linkage to systems may provide access to services and personnel otherwise unavailable.[74,75]

Along with the opportunity for growth, in many cases the institutional benefit derived is organizational survival itself. It has been noted, for example, that financial deficits, manpower shortages, and severe facilities problems have led to mergers and other types of consolidation in order to allow the institutions involved to survive.[76]

Multi-institutional systems are expected to have greater "clout" in the political arena. The strength of numbers suggest increased power for systems in relationships with external agencies, such as government, third party payers, and planning and regulatory bodies,[77] along with more influence in the local health community. This view recognizes both the political nature of hospital activity and the potential impact of a collective approach.[78]

Organizational benefits derived from the development of systems may also serve the community. Growth and expansion can improve access to care and to clinical and administrative services and programs otherwise unavailable.[79] This attribute is of particular importance to people in underserved areas. Yet another potential benefit is a broader, more com-

TABLE 3

Summary of Anticipated Benefits of
Multi-Institutional Systems

Type of Benefit	Level of Benefit	
	Institutional	**Community**

Economic	Cost savings via economies of scale
	- operating advantages, e.g.
	    increased productivity
	    improved utilization of resource
	      capacity
	    lower staffing requirements
	    reduced unit costs from joint
	      activities
	- financial advantages, e.g.
	    access to capital markets
	    improved credit standing
	    reduced borrowing costs
		lower prices
		reduced duplication
		  and excess capacity
		  of facilities
		improved resource
		  allocation

Manpower	improved recruitment of clinical
	  and management manpower
	improved retention of clinical
	  and management manpower
	strong clinical and management
	  capability
		greater access to and
		  availability of breadth
		  and depth of clinical
		  and management
		  manpower
		improved distribution
		  of health manpower

Organizational	organizational growth, e.g.
	  extend referral networks
	  penetrate new markets
	  expand existing markets
	organizational survival, e.g.
	  financial improvements
	  accreditation standards
	greater political power
		improved access to care
		increased availability
		  of services
		broader, more compre-
		  hensive scope of
		  services

prehensive range and scope of services available to the population.[80]

Thus, we see that there are economic, manpower, and organizational benefits expected from multi-institutional arrangements, at both the institutional and community levels. These anticipated benefits are summarized in Table 3. This formulation of expectations and promise provides us with a context within which to review the performance of multi-institutional systems.

The Performance of Multi-Institutional Systems

As indicated above, the performance of multi-institutional systems will be reviewed in light of their promise. The discussion will be framed in terms of the anticipated economic, manpower, and organizational benefits as they relate to the institutional and community levels. Where possible, reference will be made to particular types of inter-organizational arrangements. Finally, this review will be limited to evaluations which have taken the form of published studies, reports, or theses.

Economic Benefits

Assessment of the economic benefits of multi-institutional arrangements is the area which thus far has received the greatest attention. In a study by the Health Services Research Center of the Hospital Research and Educational Trust and Northwestern University, the programs of 16 shared service organizations were selected for evaluation.[8] Services were categorized into four groups: medical and clinical, manpower, administrative and supportive, and education and training. Four different types of structural arrangements were included: referral service, purchased or joint contract service, multisponsored service, and regional service. The effects of sharing were measured in terms of cost, accessibility, availability, comprehensiveness, quality, and acceptance. Data were collected primarily through available documentation and interviews with individuals at the study sites, through which investigators sought to assess the impact of sharing on the services involved. Analyzing the various structural arrangements, the investigators reported that results with regard to cost were generally mixed, including several instances in which the shared arrangement had an adverse effect. By type of service, improvements in costs were found among medical services. Mixed results on costs were reported for administrative and manpower services, while costs for educational services increased. Improvements were noted in quality, comprehensiveness, and access; however, the investigators concluded that to achieve these improvements, there was an increase in costs.

In another part of this study, aimed specifically at the economic impact of sharing, investigators evaluated five shared services (personnel/collective bargaining, blood banking, laundry and linen, obstetrics and pediatrics, and printing) in six case studies. Economies of scale and resultant cost savings were demonstrated, particularly in administrative services. Savings were achieved via standardization, reduced unit cost of production through increased volume of processing (laundry), and joint purchasing of blood, supplies, linen, and forms. Reduced capital requirements were reported and, where capital was needed, access to financial markets was found to be improved.

The major improvement found in medical services was in the planning, scheduling, and utilization of facilities and manpower, where the larger scale of operations achieved through sharing led to reduction in random fluctuations in demand and allowed lower reserve capacity requirements.

In an evaluation of another type of organizational arrangement, Biggs compared performance of traditionally managed nonprofit hospitals to nonprofit hospitals operating under a management contract with a for-profit corporation.[82,83] Using a matched sample of hospitals, Biggs paired traditionally managed and contract managed hospitals on the basis of number of beds, geographic location, population base, average per capita income of population, type of ownership and control, and presence of a medical education program. The matching yielded 32 pairs of hospitals, data from which were collected through a survey questionnaire.

In general, contract managed and traditionally managed hospitals appeared to be comparable. That is, within each of the parameters used for evaluation, there were more similarities than differences between the types of hospitals. There were, however, some differences of note. For example, one of the dimensions of interest in this study was economic accountability, defined in terms of the cost of hospital care. Biggs found that contract managed hospitals had a lower cost per stay than traditionally managed hospitals. While contract managed hospitals had higher per diem cost, this was offset by their shorter length of stay. The differences in cost between the hospital types, however, was not statistically significant. Contract hospitals also had fewer employees per bed, and experienced a somewhat lower proportion of total expenses devoted to payroll.

In a study of hospital mergers, Treat attempted to evaluate what he termed efficiency and effectiveness of a group of urban and rural hospitals before and after merger.[84] Efficiency measures were average cost per case, average cost per patient day, bed turnover rate, and employees per patient, while indicators of effectiveness included an index of services available, patient days, and number of approved programs. Using American Hospital Association survey data, Treat matched 32 pairs of merged with independent hospitals, using as parameters length of stay, services, geographic location, facilities, bed quantity, and number of admissions. Performance measures then were calculated for groups of paired hospitals according to size (over and under 300 beds), location (cities over and under 50,000 population), and time period (1 year before merger, and 3, 5, and 7 years after merger).

Results indicated that, among merged urban hospitals, there was an increase in service capability which was accompanied by a significant increase in cost. Thus, while patient days declined, both services and programs increased, again with a concomitant cost increase. Among merged rural hospitals, a different picture emerged, in which both effectiveness and efficiency improved. Rural mergers yielded higher occupancy, greater labor intensity, reduced length of stay, higher cost per day but lower cost per case.

Treat concluded that mergers, at least in urban areas, may not be a desirable structural alternative to improve cost efficiency and, in fact, may lead instead to diseconomies of scale.

The Samaritan Health System, based in Phoenix, Arizona, has been the subject of several evaluations. In a study by Neumann, which involved a financial analysis of the Samaritan system, it is reported that the rate of increase in the average cost per stay in the Samaritan system was not significantly different from that of a control group.[85]

Neumann indicates that while there were demonstrated cost savings, notably in support areas, these did not result in a lower average cost because of the small unaccredited hospitals in the system whose scope of services and quality were upgraded. That is, start up costs of the system and increased service capabilities, particularly the addition of services which were previously unavailable to rural areas, were responsible for the lack of visible economies. The financial advantages that did accrue spread the risk of bankruptcy over a larger asset base, stabilized the flow of funds from operations for the entire system, and provided access to external sources of capital funds to individual hospitals within the system.

An earlier evaluation of this system by Edwards and Astolfi also noted the financial advantages achieved and further stressed the start up costs and increased service capability as key factors in explaining the absence of economies of scale.[86,87,88]

A re-evaluation of the Samaritan system was part of a larger study on multihospital systems sponsored by the Hospital Research and Educational Trust in 1975.[89] Findings from this study are consistent with those of Neumann, i.e., average cost per case was greater and grew at a faster rate than that of a control group. The key factor reported to explain this finding was the cost involved in bringing the weaker hospitals in the system up to standard both financially and qualitatively.

In one of the more comprehensive studies to date, Cooney and Alexander compared the costs and revenues of eight nonprofit systems with those of a matched set of autonomous hospitals.[90,91,92] The systems ranged in size from two to seven hospitals, and in age from brand new to 12 years. The time period studied was 1967-1972. In general, seven of the eight systems proved to be cost effective when compared to the control hospitals. The system hospitals had a lower level and a slower rate of growth of average cost per case. They also showed lower gross patient revenue per stay and a slower growth rate of average gross revenue. Output of system hospitals was higher, measured as inpatient admissions adjusted for ambulatory services, despite a slower growth in bed capacity. Average length of stay was found to be lower in multihospital systems. There was also a slower growth in manhours per case. While wage rates were higher within the systems, this was not accompanied by higher labor costs.

The researchers did note immediate increases in expenses with the systems as a function of start up costs and the trauma of substantial organizational change. Over time, however, the cost situation changed in favor of the multihospital systems. Although some savings were achieved by reduction of direct expenses in clinical areas, economies of scale were most easily achieved in the hotel services. This was attributed to adaptability of labor saving technology, high utilization of bulk purchased supplies, and the lower level of conflict and absence of disputes over "turf." The reduction in manhours per case suggests greater capital intensity, more use of technology, and increased productivity within the systems. The authors speculate that the emphasis on cost control and facility utilization might be serving to encourage physicians to change their behavior and to adopt measures aimed at reducing length of stay. In one of the few direct indications of economic benefit at the community level, it is reported in this study that the savings realized were passed along to consumers in the form of lower prices.

Coyne, in a recent study, attempts to measure and determine the impact of organizational characteristics on the performance of hospitals across several types of multi-unit systems.[93] Systems were defined as three or more hospitals under the direction of a single governing board and single administration. Thus excluded were shared service organizations, consortia, and management contracts or leases. Eight nonprofit and six investor-owned systems were included, with data collected via mail questionnaire and interviews. To evaluate performance, Coyne selected average cost per patient day and occupancy as measures of efficiency.

Coyne employed a number of control variables for environmental characteristics, specifically population density, factor price differences per census region, and number of hospitals per county as an indicator of the extent of competition. For system organizational characteristics, he classified ownership as religious, other nonprofit, or investor-owned. Type of management structure, representing the division of authority and responsibility between corporate offices and hospitals, was characterized as functional, geographical, or institutional. Geographic dispersion among facilities and between facilities and corporate offices was arrayed as local, regional, multiregional, and national.

Using occupancy as the outcome measure, Coyne reports occupancy to be influenced by the type of system ownership. Religious order hospitals were found to have occupancy rates significantly higher than the other ownership types. Hospitals in geographically concentrated systems, with a high degree of centralized clinical and administrative services, were found to reduce duplication and have higher utilization than geographically dispersed systems with few centralized services. This is attributed by Coyne to patient referral networks and greater consolidation of medical staff organization.

With cost as the measure of outcome, Coyne found ownership was not associated with efficiency. Controlling for size and for organizational and environmental characteristics, costs in investor-owned hospitals were not significantly different from those in nonprofit hospitals. In highly centralized systems, the level of capital expenditure authority of the administrator was found to be associated with cost efficiency. As this authority rose from low to medium, efficiency increased; however, beyond the medium level, cost efficiency decreased. Within functionally organized systems, as geographic dispersion increased, communication and coordination problems grew and efficiency decreased. Institutionally organized systems were found to be more efficient than either functionally or geographically organized systems, leading Coyne to suggest that cost efficiency may be highest in the more autonomously structured systems.

Overall, Coyne argues that the systems owned by religious orders, institutionally structured, provide for sufficient management autonomy while retaining certain policy prerogatives in the governance function, the net result of which is greater control of costs and utilization than found in more centralized systems.

In summary, the evidence as to achievement of the anticipated economic benefits of multi-institutional arrangements appears to be mixed. At the institutional level, several studies point to increased productivity, better utilization of resource capacity, and cost-savings through joint activities. In addition, there is some evidence of reduced costs of borrowing money as a result of better credit standing. On the other hand, there is also evidence of lack of success in attaining expected economic benefits. The study on shared services reported cost increases in a number of areas. Treat's study of mergers found that, in urban mergers, utilization of resource capacity declined, productivity fell, and there was a significant increase in costs. Likewise, the studies of the Samaritan system indicate a situation of rising costs. However, in several of the studies, investigators point to improved access to care, greater availability of programs, and provision of a broader range of activities as the factors explaining the absence of economic benefits. There is presumably a trade-off made between the organizational benefit of improved service capability at the community level and economic benefit in the form of cost savings at the institutional level.

While the data on economic benefits at the institutional level are mixed, there is a general lack of evidence on economic benefits at the community level. The major exception is the Cooney and Alexander study in which lower prices were reported in multihospital systems vis-a-vis the control groups.

It must be added that the issue of whether economic benefits have been secured is confounded by methodological problems in a number of the studies. For example, findings reported in the study of 16 shared services organizations were based on limited documentation and on individual perceptions of the impact of sharing. Detailed cost data generally were not available, restricting the rigor of the analysis. In some cases, the outcome measures employed may be suspect. For instance, it is not clear that cost per patient day is an appropriate measure of "cost efficiency." Another complicating factor is the potential change in the mix of resources used and the product mix as a result of multi-institutional arrangement. These factors, as well as the case mix, may vary, thereby confounding the analysis. That is, in the absence of control factors to assure that we are measuring the same phenomena, it is difficult to discern if indeed economies of scale have been achieved.

Manpower Benefits

Manpower benefits at the institutional level concern the recruitment and retention of both clinical and management personnel. Only some of the studies explicitly address this issue. Treat, for instance, found that rural hospitals which merged improved their ability to recruit personnel.[94] Cooney and Alexander reported that although the Samaritan system devoted substantial effort to recruitment of physicians for the rural hospitals, there was only modest success. Further, there continued to be problems of retention.[95] At the community level, the studies of the Samaritan Health System indicate that the rural hospitals in that system did indeed benefit from the availability of management and clinical consultation services and from educational programs.[96] This additional specialized personnel was seen as instrumental in upgrading the quality in the rural hospitals served by the Samaritan system.

It is reasonably clear that many systems have been able to attract and retain management personnel. Cooney and Alexander, in their study of a number of systems, reported on issues in the use of such talent.[97] Based upon discussions with administrative personnel within 16 systems, they found that a hospital based administrative staff was viewed as the preferred structure for local systems of up to four or five hospitals. Beyond these parameters, the corporate staff structure was preferred. Such a corporate staff offered the advantages of providing specialized expertise in areas to which hospital based staff could not attend. This expertise could also be shared across hospitals in the system. There were noted difficulties with corporate staff, however, such as their tendency to over-control member hospitals, to limit local decision making, and to slow the decision making through added approval requirements. Across the systems, there may exist problems between corporate and hospital staff of lack of a uniform perspective or understanding of their respective roles within the system.

To summarize, the data provide some support for the expectation of improved recruitment and retention of personnel. In several instances, multihospital systems and their individual institutions were found to have secured manpower benefits, although physician recruitment and retention continues to be a matter of concern. The anticipated benefits of specialized management capability have, to a large extent, been realized for the systems and member institutions, but problems of interrelationships apparently require attention. The communities served by multi-institutional systems appear to be benefiting, quantitatively and qualitatively, from the availability of specialized clinical and managerial talent.

Organizational Benefits

The evidence to date would indicate that a number of the expected benefits at the institutional level have been achieved. In the studies of the Samaritan system, it was reported that the organizational survival of several urban and rural hospitals was a result of joining this multihospital system.[98,99] The hospitals involved benefited in terms of financial capability, operating systems improvements, and a greater ability to meet accreditation and licensure standards. It is quite clear that organizational growth has occurred, and that markets and service areas have been expanded. As part of their study, Cooney and Alexander reviewed some of the issues related to organizational growth via formation of multi-institutional arrangements.[100,101] Their analysis included 16 multihospital systems, ranging from a two hospital satellite system to a multistate system of over 80 hospitals. Involved were systems both old and new, large and small, nonprofit and investor-owned, interstate and regional. The systems represented were from urban as well as rural environments. Structurally, there were instances of merged and mixed governing boards, combined and autonomous medical staffs, and centralized and decentralized operating management responsibilities. To gather the requisite data, administrative personnel from the systems were asked for their perceptions of the organization and the environment.

In general, findings showed that systems operating six or more hospitals tended to be more structured and formalized, but were perceived as less effective in accomplishing tasks and achieving organizational goals. Older systems, seven years and over, were seen as being less formalized, better able to cope with the environment, having superior organizational communication and coordination, and were generally more effective in accomplishing goals and tasks. Thus, it was suggested that the benefits attributed to organizational growth and expansion might be constrained by the size of the organization and may require substantial time to achieve.

At the community level, the study of shared services revealed that, across the types of arrangements, quality of services along with the comprehensiveness of and accessibility to services were perceived to have improved.[102] In terms of the types of services (medical, administrative, eductional, and manpower), quality was seen as the most improved factor, followed by comprehensiveness. Quality and comprehensiveness and, to a lesser extent, access were the most consistently reported areas of improvement resulting from shared services. It must be reiterated, however, that these improvements were accompanied by increases in cost. Further, the researchers noted problems relevant to access, as a result of resource reallocation and transportation difficulties.

Biggs, in his study comparing contract managed with traditionally managed hospitals, reported a different result. He found few significant differences in terms of services and programs offered, facilities and manpower available, or the resultant quality (with the exception of a higher consultation rate in contract managed hospitals).[103]

Biggs also explored the nature of the relationships, which he termed social accountability, between the hospitals and their various constituencies. He found that contract managed hospitals were more likely to use the media to inform their communities about hospital activities, and were significantly higher in the use of questionnaires for discharged patients to evaluate their hospitalization. Biggs suggested that contract managed hospitals appeared to be somewhat more aggressive in developing strategies to deal with their environment and to relate to their communities.

As noted earlier, Treat, in his evaluation of mergers, found increased service capability in both urban and rural hospitals.[104] In the studies of the Samaritan Health System, findings consistently showed community-level benefits in terms of increased comprehensiveness, access, and availability of services.[105,106] It was argued that these benefits served to improve the quality of care offered to people in the rural areas.

In the Cooney and Alexander study of the Samaritan system, organizational growth was found to result in a greater number of services becoming available to the service population of the rural hospitals.[107] It was noted, however, that the delivery site for many of the services was not the rural hospital itself but rather was through referral arrangement to the larger urban hospitals in the system.

Overall, the studies suggest that expected organizational benefits at the institutional level have been realized. Evidence has been presented to indicate organizational survival and organizational growth. While increased political power has been suggested as an organizational benefit, there does not yet appear to be empirical evidence to assess. At the community level, several of the studies point to achievement of improved access to care, greater availability of care, and a broadened range and scope of hospital services for the people served by multi-institutional systems. It has been presumed that the improvements, along with structural changes made within the affiliated organizations, have served to enhance the quality of care provided.

Summary

On balance, one of the more consistent findings in these evaluations lies in the organizational benefits of improved access, availability and scope of hospital services for those in previously underserved areas. Benefiting particularly are rural institutions experiencing operating deficiencies, and their service populations. That these benefits often have been accompanied by increases in costs should not be surprising. To the extent that many interorganizational arrangements have as an objective increased service capability, it would not be unreasonable to expect concomitant increases in cost. A key problem noted earlier, however, is that since the resource and product mix may well have changed, we do not know if such increases are in fact concomitant.

Manpower benefits have received relatively modest attention in these studies. It is evident that management capability has been enhanced. While some success in the recruitment and retention of clinical personnel has been reported, there remain difficulties in this area.

The evidence as to achievement of economic benefit is mixed, at best. Those economic benefits reported are primarily in the hotel and support service areas, where labor saving technology is easily applied and where turf disputes are minimized. The Cooney and Alexander study provides the most positive findings thus far with regard to cost savings, but it does reemphasize the need to allow sufficient time for economic benefits to accrue.[108] While savings have been reported in the administrative areas, there would appear to be far greater potential through integration of patient care and medical service areas.[109,110] Generally, however, such integration has not been very widespread and is perhaps most applicable at the local or regional level where markets can be restructured.[111]

While multi-institutional arrangements have shown dramatic growth, now representing a significant portion of the hospital industry, there is available relatively little research or evaluation. Reviewing the anticipated benefits, several important areas of interest still require assessment. For example, economic benefits at the community level remain largely unexplored and manpower benefits have had but limited attention. The conditions under which increased service capability (quantitative and qualitative) offset achievement of economic benefit, and the long-run impact of such a trade-off is a central policy issue which must be addressed. Further, the implications of different types of organizational arrangements with regard to their impact on the achievement of economic, manpower, and organizational benefits merit significantly greater investigation.

Among the studies reviewed, problems of the measures used and potential changes of resource, case, and product mix have been noted. Some of the samples have limited generalizability and several studies are cross-sectional and do not account for changes over time. Indeed, Studnicki has suggested that multihospital systems per se are perhaps too broad and complex a concept for explaining changes in outcomes; rather what is needed is greater specificity and selectivity among the units of analysis.[112]

The work done thus far offers us a beginning as we attempt to understand the dynamics and the impact of interorganizational arrangements. However, we still lack a substantial body of empirical evidence on the real and total effects of organizational integration. While some of the anticipated benefits have been realized, and while the promise is significant indeed, there remains much to be done by way of determining the relationship between that promise and the performance of multi-institutional systems.

Barriers to Multi-Institutional Systems

As we attempt to assess the performance of multi-institutional arrangements in light of their promise, it becomes clear that a number of environmental barriers exist that serve to impede their development and the realization of potential benefits. While a variety of forces have operated to encourage their formation and growth, at the same time there are countervailing forces. In the legal area, especially antitrust and tax laws, and in the financial area, particularly in reimbursement mechanisms, a number of developments appear to be moving in quite a different direction, serving to constrain interinstitutional arrangements and thus preclude or dampen the achievement of their objectives.*

Antitrust

Antitrust laws, notably the Sherman and Clayton Acts, are designed to preserve and promote free competition within the economy. In general, these laws apply to two areas: *anticompetitive conduct* (e.g., price fixing, territorial division, boycotts) and *anticompetitive structures* (e.g., mergers, expansion, integration of organizations).

To this point, the hospital industry has not been exempted from the application of the antitrust laws and a series of recent court actions would indicate that hospitals in general and multi-institutional systems in particular may be subject to the restrictions of the antitrust laws. Many activities of these systems could be construed to constitute anticompetitive behavior and one must conclude that, regardless of the motive for the behavior, prosecution is possible. Drawing on a recent review of this situation,[113] examples of activities where hospitals and multiple hospital systems may be vulnerable are summarized below:

1. Hospital mergers which "substantially lessen competition or create a monopoly" may be in violation of Section VII of the Clayton Act. Hospitals in a close geographical area which are contemplating merger as the means of integration (regardless of the intent) face possible civil suit.

---

* Much of the material in the following three sections is adapted from Vraciu, R.A., and Zuckerman, H.S. "Legal and Financial Constraints on the Development and Growth of Multiple Hospital Arrangements," *Health Care Management Review*, Winter 1979, Aspen Systems Corporation, Germantown, MD.

On this issue, Starkweather, Greenawalt, and Mehringer have noted that the concern of the Justice Department revolves around high or increasing concentration or domination in a local market.[114] This concern with the nature of the market is of particular interest to local or regional systems, serving a geographically defined population. Urban hospital mergers or consortia, for example, might be especially vulnerable. National or multiregional systems, such as the investor-owned or religious order chains, may not be similarly affected.[115]

2. Sharing budgets and discussions of prices by hospitals under separate corporate ownership could constitute price fixing prohibited under the Sherman Act.

3. "Cooperative attempts" by hospitals to divide markets through the allocation of customers among themselves could be illegal under the Sherman Act. Thus, efforts to reduce duplication of services and match the capacity of hospitals with expected demand, might be considered illegal as an unreasonable restriction of competition.

One of the key community level objectives of several types of multi-institutional arrangements, the rationalization of planning in order to overcome the problems of duplication and excess capacity, may be vulnerable under this interpretation.

4. Multiple hospital system arrangements which represent a substantial portion of providers in a particular geographical area might be charged with conspiring to restrict the supply of hospital services in a noncompetitive way or to be attempting to obtain monopoly power. Efforts to prevent outsiders from establishing themselves in the market could be viewed as violations of the Sherman Act.

In the *Hospital Building Company v. Trustees of Rex Hospital* case, the parties were said to be conspiring to control the bed supply, blocking relocation and expansion of a for-profit hospital, and were generally restraining the business of providing hospital services, all of this via blocking authorization under certificate-of-need procedures. It has been argued that this control of the market place is, of course, one of the purposes for which many multihospital systems are designed.[116] In addition, laid to rest in this case was the notion that hospitals are not involved in interstate commerce and thus are not liable under antitrust law.[117,118,119] Evidence of the purchase of supplies and medicine from out-of-state sellers, out-of-state patients, revenue from out-of-state insurance companies and federal governmental programs, management contract fees paid to an out-of-state based corporation, and expansion plans to be financed by out-of-state lenders led the U.S. Supreme Court to rule that interstate commerce was indeed involved.

In a recent action, a federal district court in Detroit dismissed an antitrust suit brought by a Michigan corporation which had been denied a certificate-of-need to build a new hospital (*Huron Valley Hospital, Inc. v. City of Pontiac*).[120,121] Shortly thereafter, an existing hospital received approval to replace its facility, leading Huron Valley to charge that there existed a conspiracy to restrain market entry. In dismissing the case, the judge concluded that Congress intended to grant health systems agencies exemption from antitrust laws. However, this case, now under appeal, does not address the scope of such exemption, thus its possible application to private planning by hospital and hospital systems is unclear.

The potential for suit or prosecution, and the attendant costs, may serve as a barrier to multi-institutional systems. Court action may be initiated by regulatory agencies or by other providers who see their interests adversely affected by the growth and development of systems. Further, the antitrust laws are not neutral to organizational forms. That is, multiple hospital systems with separate ownership and centralized management control appear more vulnerable to legal challenge than systems with decentralized management control; and hospital systems in geographic proximity are more vulnerable than are systems which are geographically dispersed.[122]

Antitrust law is premised on the notion that competition is inherently good and monopolistic behavior is inherently bad. This dichotomy avoids the issue of whether competition in the health field, given its market imperfection, better serves the public interest than does cooperative behavior.

The matter of the public interest is perhaps the issue around which the planning/antitrust contradiction will be resolved. The test may well be whether organizational integrations *unreasonably* restrain trade. The questions involved relate to the effects on the public interest of restricting competition, whether integration yields results favorable to the public interest, and whether the public benefits of consolidation exceed the costs of restricting competition.

Federal Tax Laws

Federal tax laws have served to penalize certain types of multi-institutional arrangements by taxing income. For the most part, the laws constrain shared services among organizations retaining separate ownership. The tax consequences of establishing shared services organizations have been analyzed by Bromberg[123,124] and recently were sum-

marized as follows:[125]
1. There are restrictions on the types of services eligible for sharing. A shared service organization established as a 501(e) organization–both tax exempt and eligible for tax deductible donations–is limited to providing certain enumerated services, of which laundry services has been clearly omitted.

However, a U.S. District Court recently ruled that a centralized laundry, operated by six nonprofit hospitals, could not be denied tax exempt status.[126] The Court concluded that although laundry services were not listed in Section 501(e), the intent was to expand, not limit, cooperative services. Further, the Court ruled that the joint laundry did not lose charitable status simply because it offered services provided by commercial organizations. Finally, shared laundry services which were viewed as essential, realizing no profit and operating exclusively for the benefit of tax exempt hospitals, could not reasonably be defined as unrelated trade or business. This ruling, if upheld upon appeal, would remove one of the barriers to shared services.
2. There are also restrictions on the membership of shared services organizations. Shared service organizations established under 501(e) can provide services only to governmental hospitals and to other nonprofit organizations established under 501(c)(3). Thus, investor-owned hospitals and tax exempt nursing homes could not receive services from a Section 501(e) organization. A shared service organization established under 501(c)(3) may provide services to for-profit hospitals only to the extent that these remain an insubstantial part of the overall activities of the organization.
3. The payout or allocation requirements of Section 501(e) and Subchapter T (Non-Exempt Cooperative) shared services organizations can lead to capital problems for the shared services organization and/or liquidity problems for the hospitals.

While these cooperatives can render services to nonmember organizations and are free of restrictions on the kinds of services provided, they must pay out or allocate all net earnings to avoid corporate taxation, thus leading to adverse reimbursement consequences and limiting the accumulation of cash reserves.
4. Shared service organizations established under 501(c)(3) have no such payout requirements, do not limit type of service to be shared, and are eligible for tax deductible donations. This type of status allows the organization to maintain the cash flow necessary to build up capital reserves. The major difficulty arises in obtaining such

status. The Internal Revenue Service has taken the position that a shared service organization cannot qualify under this section unless it qualifies under the provision of Section 501(e). While the federal courts have held against this overly restrictive interpretation, hospitals seeking this status are nevertheless required to work through the courts—a time consuming and costly effort.

5. The tax treatment of "unrelated business taxable income" earned by one hospital selling services to another hospital or health care provider limits the desirability of this kind of shared service arrangement. Although the "economies of scale" argument can be made for many direct sales arrangements, services cannot be sold to nonhospitals or to hospitals with more that 100 beds, at a rate in excess of cost, unless the hospital selling the services is willing to pay income tax on the proceeds. Moreover, the services can only be sold to tax exempt and governmental hospitals.

Overall, restrictions on tax exempt status, types of services and hospitals eligible for sharing, payout provisions, and the taxability of specific categories of income, serve as barriers to the development of shared services, thereby limiting the ability to accrue the benefits associated with such cooperative activities. The Internal Revenue Code and IRS do not prevent shared services arrangements per se, but rather they pose obstacles which appear inconsistent with the mandate of P. L. 93-641.

Reimbursement

Existing reimbursement mechanisms fail to provide incentives for and often serve as constraints upon the growth and development of multi-institutional arrangements. Reimbursement consequences are perhaps greatest in the areas of accumulation of capital and reimbursement for operating expenses.

Capital Requirements

Organizations need an inflow of funds corresponding to total financial requirements, i.e., current operating needs plus capital requirements. Capital needs of hospitals include working capital and plant capital to replace existing facilities and equipment and to add new technology. The development and expansion of multi-unit organizations often necessitate significant funds to finance their activities.[127] For instance, when two or more physically deteriorated and/or financially troubled hospitals merge, capital for a new facility may be necessary. Shared service organizations, set up as separate corporations, often require start-up and expansion capital.

The Medicare reimbursement formula, however, does not allow a contribution to capital for nonprofit hospitals. Such hospitals have moved toward greater use of debt financing as philanthropy as a source of capital funds has declined and the base of charge-paying patients has decreased.[128] Since nonprofit multihospital systems operate in the same environment, these systems must face a choice between a high debt position and restrictions on growth potential. Particularly affected are those institutions with high percentage Medicare/Medicaid business which may recognize the need for integration with other organizations, but may be unable to generate the start-up capital necessary for any number of forms of consolidation.

For-profit hospitals clearly are favored in Medicare reimbursement as they receive a source of capital unavailable to not-for-profit hospitals. That is, for-profit or investor-owned hospitals are allowed a return on equity, at least a portion of which generally is retained to meet capital needs.[129] In addition, the ability to sell stock offers yet another source of capital.

There are indications that some of the existing disincentives in Medicare reimbursement regulation may be removed. For example, the Health Care Financing Administration recently proposed to reimburse hospitals at the billed charge for services obtained from a *related* shared services organization if the charges do not exceed the market price for comparable services.[130] This will enable shared services organizations to accumulate some of the capital necessary for working capital needs and growth. Such reimbursement is currently based on costs and capital must be accumulated strictly from patients and third parties paying on the basis of charges. However, a more stringent definition of *related* organization may serve to offset the removal of the disincentive.

Several suggestions have been made for improvements in the area of capital requirements. For example, it has been argued that multi-institutional systems offer potential advantages in capital formation, accumulation, and allocation.[131,132] Systems could be allowed to pool depreciation funds among member hospitals, to be used to support needed renovation, construction, or equipment. Such an arrangement would provide flexibility in allocating resources within a system, supporting services among the units and funding new and diversified services needed medically and geographically.

Intrasystem borrowing or lending might be used to reduce the need for and higher cost of external financing. Such internal cross subsidization would aid overall system financial stability. Interest expenses for intrasystem borrowing is not now an allowable cost (except in religious order systems), yet the cost of borrowing is allowed if provided through an external organization, often at higher interest rates.[133]

In summary, it would appear that a number of modifications in reimbursement policy related to capital requirements could serve to remove disincentives, add positive incentives, and aid multi-institutional systems to achieve their potential.

Operating Expenses

There are several areas where multiple hospital systems are adversely affected by reimbursement for operating expenses. An example is the "pay out provision" for shared services organizations established under 501(e), requiring that such organizations distribute the net earnings to their patrons.[134] Since these organizations require capital of their own, the distribution of earnings often is in the form of scrip, thus providing no cash to the hospital. Medicare reimbursement regulations treat this scrip as an offset to the allowable costs of the purchased services, potentially decreasing the hospital's liquidity position.

Another area is Medicare's limiting its liability to hospital routine service costs according to a particular hospital's relationship to a "peer group" determined by hospital bed size and location.[135] Hospitals above the 80th percentile of their peer group are reimbursed at the 80th percentile. A single hospital within a multiple hospital system may offer a more sophisticated set of services and treat a more complex case mix than independent hospitals of the same size by virtue of its ties with other hospitals in the system. Consequently, a hospital in a multiple hospital system may lie at the high end of the distribution and be penalized because of its shared clinical services arrangements.

A number of other reimbursement issues are problematic for multi-institutional systems. Within Catholic systems, lay equivalent salaries are reimbursable only if incurred in individual facilities, and are not allowable if incurred in the corporate office.[136] Medicare requirements to file individual hospital balance sheets ignore those systems which have consolidated assets into a single organization with a combined balance sheet.[137] Further, Medicare has discouraged the development of self-insurance plans by limiting or denying reimbursement of expenses under such plans. This is particularly damaging to multihospital systems which have led in developing such plans and have large insured populations over which to spread the risk.[138] Self-insurance programs developed by multihospital systems have been reported to result in reduced malpractice insurance outlays, with rates substantially lower on a per bed basis than charges from commercial carriers for the same coverage.[139]

For purposes of reimbursement it has been suggested that systems might be treated as combined entities, rather than individual institutions, thus allowing internal reallocation of reimbursement dollars within the system.[140] Provider certification rules under Medicare, however, allow for an entity with multiple components to be treated as a single provider only under certain conditions. The organizations involved must: (a) be subject to the control and direction of one governing body; (b) have a single chief medical officer who reports to the governing body and is responsible for all medical staff activities in all components; (c) show total integration of the medical staff by credentialing them without limitation to all components, and by having committees responsible for specific areas of concern in all components of the hospital; and (d) have a single chief executive officer to whom all administrative authority flows and who can exercise administrative control over all components.[141] While the virtues of internal reallocation may be debated, the current regulations serve to encourage certain kinds of organizational consolidations but is not responsive to alternative structures.

Current capital and operating reimbursement policies constrain the growth and development of multi-institutional systems and thus impede their ability to achieve the potential benefits.

Organizational Constraints

In addition to environmental factors, there are forces operating within institutions and their communities which may serve as barriers to the growth and development of interinstitutional arrangements. Among these are concerns related to loss of institutional identity and autonomy, fear of domination, uncertainty as to role changes, and imbalances in power which may lead to inequities in resource allocation.

At the outset, it should be recognized that the movement toward multihospital systems suggests a change in values. Historically, hospitals have competed for resources, for patients, and for physicians. Pressure to shift from competition and autonomy to a mode marked by cooperation, sharing, and joint activity is indeed a new direction and represents a different value set.[142] In addition, an underlying assumption in this process is that the key actors will act rationally, will be willing to place community welfare above institutional concerns, and can convince other key actors in the organizational power structure to do the same.[143]

These organizational and community factors undoubtedly have influenced the rate of growth of multi-institutional systems, the strategies employed to market such systems, and the organizational forms that systems have adopted. For example, in describing the recently developed Maryland Health Care System, McDaniel emphasizes the need to preserve the relative independence of member institutions.[144] In attempting to gain the requisite support of trustees, physicians, and managers, the arguments used for cooperation focused on the notion that voluntary association among independent entities would serve to strengthen each members' position in its own community by expanding its expertise and its capability to deal with the various sociological, professional, technological, economic, and political pressures. In the formation of this system, hospitals were sought as members if their services would be complementary rather than duplicative, thereby identifying noncompetitive markets. The development of particular kinds of organizational forms, such as consortia and management contracts are, in large part, mechanisms designed to overcome concerns over autonomy and control while pursuing the advantages of consolidation.[145,146]

Trustee concerns regarding the status and authority of the local board within a multi-institutional system, relationship of the local board to the corporate board, changing roles and responsibilities of trustees, and potential loss of status and prestige are among the issues raised in the development of systems.[147,148] Overall, it is clear that trustee reaction to participation in multi-organizational systems, and the attendant fears and doubts, is a powerful force and a potential barrier.

Physician response also may serve as an inhibiting force to interorganizational activity. Questions regarding staff privileges, relationships with physicians in other hospitals in the system, proposed peer review activities, implications for existing clinical and financial arrangements with the local hospital, impact on practice patterns and patient referral networks, and effect on status in the professional community represent some of the areas of physician concern.[149,150]

In addition to trustees and physicians, hospital managers may be a source of opposition to interorganizational arrangements. Concern over job status and security, and a view that integrative efforts may reflect negatively on administrative performance have been cited as barriers to system development.[151] In addition, managers may share with trustees and physicians the apprehension over loss of local control and autonomy.

The concerns of trustees, physicians, administrators, along with those of other personnel within the institutions involved, represent a nontrivial problem. The trauma involved in organizational consolidation, and the impact on achieving the benefits of interinstitutional arrangements was highlighted by the Cooney and Alexander study.[152] Attention has been drawn to the process by which such arrangements evolve and to the importance of understanding and dealing with the behavioral implications of integration.[153,154] The need for clarification of roles and expectations, and for explicit discussion of the organizational transition have been identified as essential to overcoming barriers to system development.[155,156]

Thus, there is a set of organizational constraints, revolving about issues of values, attitudes, and roles, which should be recognized and addressed as we seek to secure the benefits of interorganizational arrangements.

Opportunities for Further Development

In the preceding section, it was noted that a number of barriers exist which serve to constrain the achievement of the promise of multi-institutional arrangements. Beyond these barriers, however, there are several areas which multi-institutional systems themselves may explore in an effort to more fully realize their potential.

Horizontal and Vertical Integration

The literature on multi-institutional systems generally characterizes the forms of organizational integration as either horizontal or vertical.[157,158] Horizontal integration refers to the linkage of similar organizations which are at the same stage of the production process, exemplified by aggregations among and between hospitals. Vertical integration refers to linkages of organizations at immediately related stages of the production and distribution process, which may be illustrated by aggregations of hospitals with nursing homes, ambulatory care centers, and health maintenance organizations.[159]

It has been noted that many of the existing integrative arrangements are horizontal in nature, linking hospitals to other hospitals within corporately structured management systems, designed to secure economic benefits and to confront external pressures.[160] These horizontally integrated systems, which may be geographically proximate or dispersed, are seen as advantageous at the institutional level in acquiring critical resources and in coping with managerial and financial deficiencies. Community level benefits achieved thus far have tended to concentrate around hospital oriented services.

Vertically integrated multi-institutional systems, however, may offer potential which includes not only institutional advantages but also moves extensively into community benefits. Connors, for example, argues that systems could be vehicles for fundamental changes in the delivery of health services.[161] He suggests that systems should be concerned with the development of coordinated, comprehensive plans of services for their communities, plans which would include various types and levels of care and which would involve linkages with other providers and agencies. Farley contends that systems are in a unique position to use their capabilities to alter the mechanisms for delivery of care to achieve what have been defined here as community as well as institutional benefits.[162] Toomey also claims that vertically integrated systems are important to secure community level benefits. He describes the Greenville system as one moving from a comprehensive institutionally focused system toward provision of medical care services in the context of community oriented programs, extending into homes, offices, and industry, and including personal, community, and institutional services along with medical and health education programs.[163,164]

These views suggest a broad perspective as to the future role of multihospital systems. Implicit in this formulation is the notion that clinical as well as management services be integrated and that linkages with other health, social, and educational agencies be established. Such efforts could lead, as Sigmond has pointed out, to increased responsibilities for systems in the context of health delivery for a geographically defined population.[165]

Thus, vertical integration may offer opportunities for systems to provide greater access to and availability of services and manpower, along with increases in comprehensiveness and continuity of care. Further, by including alternatives to hospital care, such systems could serve to reduce excess hospital capacity and to influence costs of care to the population served. For the most part, however, strategies to develop vertically integrated systems have not been widely demonstrated. The challenge, as Stull sees it, is how to move the enlightened self-interest and creative entrepreneurship which has marked the development of most systems toward an orientation focusing on vertical as well as horizontal integration.[166]

Academic Health Centers

As discussed above, one of the perceived benefits of multi-institutional arrangements is the recruitment and retention of clinical manpower. One could argue that this benefit might be more easily attained were there closer interrelationships between multi-institutional systems, which have evolved largely around consolidation for delivery of services, and academic health centers, whose primary focus lies in the production and distribution of health manpower.

To date, there is relatively little evidence of systems working in conjunction with academic health centers. Levitan has noted that joint effort may be precluded by differences in mission.[167] The primary objectives of academic health centers are education and research, with service of interest to the extent that it supports the educational mission. Further, teaching hospitals may be large enough already to take advantage of economies of scale, and it is not clear that yet larger scale would lead to greater benefit clinically, organizationally, or politically. On the other hand, linkages between systems and academic centers could be mutually advantageous. The academic center may benefit through programs for students, interns, and residents at community hospitals, educational opportunities for faculty at affiliated hospitals, and from availability of the management capability of the multihospital systems.[168,169] Systems may benefit from access to a variety of clinical manpower resources to serve their populations and from continuing education programs for local physicians.[170] In turn, communities can benefit from greater access to and availability of highly trained clinical manpower. The mechanisms to achieve integration may, in some instances, involve coordination between academic health centers and multihospital systems. In other instances, the academic centers may attempt to create their own systems. A case in point is the Rush-Presbyterian-St. Luke's network.[171,172] This system serves over one and one-half million people in both urban and rural areas as well as producing and distributing physicians and other health manpower. The network offers various practice experiences in different settings to students, thus using network institutions for training purposes while serving as a source of needed manpower to these institutions. Plans for the system include development of continuing professional education programs, ambulatory care programs, shared services, and management contract arrangements.

In a project recently funded by the W. K. Kellogg Foundation, Boston University Hospitals seeks to develop management contracts with community hospitals and ambulatory care centers in the Boston area and to demonstrate the role of an academic health center in developing a comprehensive, vertically integrated system.[173] It is hoped that one result will be a teaching network for the medical center, involving strong educational relationships with those hospitals managed by contract. It is anticipated that clinical and professional services, based at Boston University Hospital, will be shared and certain specialized tertiary care services will be decentralized to the managed facilities.

To some extent, the growth of systems represents entry into areas historically the sole domain of academic centers, thus there is potential for a competitive posture.[174] There may be difficulties in terms of conflicting objectives, differing governance and medical staff structures, and differences in financing mechanisms. On balance, however, the benefits to the community and to the organizations involved would appear to outweigh the risks. Warden has concluded that through such interrelationships, continuing education for professionals could improve, a greater diversity of clinical experiences for students could be provided through a broadened range of facilities, services, and patients, and new referral networks could be developed.[175] At the community level, such linkages could serve to rationalize the production and distribution of health manpower, provide a mechanism to regionalize services with different levels of care, and improve access to manpower resources and services. Thus, linkage between multi-institutional systems and academic health centers may well be a significant step in achieving the expected manpower benefits.

Management and Governance

In addition to coordination of the production and distribution of clinical health manpower, it is also necessary to assure that administrative manpower is adequate to enable the achievement of the benefits of multi-institutional arrangements. Indeed, the success of systems is premised heavily on strong management capabilities.[176,177,178]

The very notion of multi-institutional systems suggest cooperation, integration, and an orientation toward balancing the needs of individual organizations with those of the system. To a large extent, however, education and training have focused on preparing individuals to be managers in autonomous, freestanding facilities in which policy making occurs at the individual institutional level.[179] The movement toward integrated systems may mean significant changes in the role of the manager and in the organizational environment in which the manager works.

Future managers should be familiar with the various types of multi-institutional arrangements, the circumstances and conditions under which the alternative forms develop, the organizational dynamics of systems, and the likely impact of these arrangements. The very nature of multi-institutional systems would seem to indicate a need for emphasis not only on *intra*organizational but on *inter*organizational theory and behavior as well. By definition, systems involve growing interaction among hospitals and between hospitals and other health agencies. Managers within these systems will increasingly be involved in interorganizational activities and processes.[180,181] Concern for and understanding of the external environment is further necessitated by increased regulatory control, consumer demands, and greater accountability. As resource allocation decisions are further influenced by external forces, Brown notes that managers must be able to coalesce various interests within the organization in order to deal effectively with agencies outside the organization.[182] Thus, growing organizational interdependency, operating in a more complex technical and behavioral environment, may well mean new and expanded roles for managers and, as Shortell points out, "will require new ways of thinking about the management process in health services organizations."[183]

In addition to changes in the role of the generalist manager, the corporate structure of multi-institutional systems may require the development of management specialists in various functional areas. Such "functional specialists" would likely have training in health administration, but would concentrate in a functional area such as finance, operations research, marketing, planning, or human resources management. Individuals so trained could work in a staff capacity at the corporate level, combining specialized knowledge with an understanding of health care organizations. Further, career mobility to positions at the institutional level need not be precluded.

To meet the managerial requirements of multi-institutional systems, attention should not be focused solely on those preparing to enter the field. There is, in addition, the need to assure managerial competence on a continuing basis for those already located in multi-institutional organizations. A number of professional organizations, such as the American College of Hospital Administrators, the American Hospital Association, and the Hospital Financial Management Association, will likely bear major responsibility in this area. University based programs in health and hospital administration also could serve as a resource for the continuing education of system managers. Further, since the corporate level staffs of multi-institutional systems are often discipline or functionally trained, the university based programs could assist in providing broadly based educational programs to orient these managers to the various facets of the health care industry. Several of the systems themselves are becoming active in continuing education for their management staffs. For example, through its Center for Health Studies, the Hospital Corporation of America is developing educational programs for hospital and corporate level management staff.[184] The focus in these programs is on financial management, human resources management, leadership, and management systems. There is also an advanced program in multiple facilities management aimed at preparing individuals to move to regional or corporate management.

Thus, to assure continued managerial competence in an increasingly complex environment, various educational alternatives might be explored. These involve reconsideration of the role of the manager in the context of multi-institutional systems, the potential for functional specialists, and the need for continuing management education.

Along with the need for continuing management capability, securing the benefits of systems will require attention to the function of governance. Coyne, in his study, noted the critical importance of the governance function on the performance of hospitals in multi-institutional systems.[185] As systems continue to evolve, it is argued that trustees will have to focus on long-range planning and strategic decision making, while moving away from involvement in institutional operations.[186] The governance role in these emerging organizations requires individuals who can work as part and think in terms of systems.[187] Trustees will be charged to make difficult resource allocation decisions, attempting to balance the needs of the system with those of the individual facilities.[188] Trustees at the corporate level are encouraged to think in terms of the greatest good for the entire system. At the local level, trustees seek to protect their hospitals for their communities, while attempting to view their facilities within the context of a network of institutions.

As part of a major organizational restructuring, the Sisters of Mercy Health Corporation is devoting substantial time and attention to the governance function.[189,190] Efforts are being made to enhance the capability of governance at the local level through changes in board composition, new educational programs, and by providing greater clarity as to roles and responsibilities. In addition, the linkage between local and corporate governance is being strengthened.

Improving the capability of the governance function is a crucial task as systems seek to achieve their potential. Education for trustees in multi-institutional settings is taking on new importance, and programs must be designed to assure adequate understanding of the changing, challenging environment in which trustees will be working.

Summary and Conclusions

The evidence to date indicates clearly that the hospital industry is evolving from a set of rather independent facilities to a mode of highly interdependent, multi-institutional organizations. These emerging organizations, which have assumed a variety of forms, offer substantial promise to their communities and to the institutions themselves in terms of economic, manpower, and organizational benefits. The achievement of these benefits has, to some extent, been constrained by a number of environmental and organizational barriers. In addition, there are important areas of activity yet to be explored by the systems in order to more fully realize their potential.

Over time, it is expected that there will be continued development and growth of multi-institutional systems. Pluralism will likely continue to characterize the ownership, financing, and operating approaches of systems. However, as external pressures mount to control costs and reduce capacity, the predominant patterns may be those which include ownership obligations and tighter management arrangements. It seems quite possible that organizations gradually will move toward more pervasive types of consolidations. Indeed, arrangements such as shared services and consortia may serve to create an environment within which organizations begin to develop more far-reaching and extensive degrees of integration.

As systems grow, it is likely that we shall witness continued interaction and cooperative activity among these organizations, evidence of which is already beginning to accumulate. Yet, at the same time, there will be increased competition among and between systems. Indication of competition between investor-owned and not-for-profit systems already is being evidenced. In addition, as nonprofit systems continue to expand, there may arise intersystem competition for manpower resources, new markets, access to capital, and technology.

Continuing consolidation and organizational integration will bring greater concentration of economic and political power. While this concentration holds great promise, there are probably limits to the degree of concentration appropriate to the public interest. This means constant vigilance to balance the needs of multi-institutional systems with those of the communities and people served. Thoughtful observers of the multihospital movement have raised a number of public policy questions in this regard.[191,192] They ask if systems will be responsive to community needs, if access to care can be balanced against the need to reduce capacity, if cost savings will be passed on to consumers, if community demands can be reconciled with system needs, and if the desire for organizational growth and new technology will conflict with efforts for planning and cost control.

These issues bring us full circle. We have described a range of organizational arrangements, emanating largely from within the hospital industry, designed to deal with the very public policy questions raised. We have seen that these arrangements hold substantial promise to the communities served as well as to the organizations themselves. We have seen that while some of the promise has been fulfilled, there remains much to be done. It has been shown that constraints such as antitrust, tax law, reimbursement policies, and organizational barriers have served to preclude the realization of the potential of multi-institutional systems. It has also been noted that there are avenues yet to be pursued by the systems themselves. These interorganizational arrangements represent not only a reconfiguration of the hospital industry, but further suggest that systems may assume new roles and broadened responsibilities. To meet these responsibilities, and to fulfill these roles, systems may move toward greater clinical as well as management integration, and develop stronger interrelationships with those organizations involved with the production and distribution of clinical and administrative manpower. As this process evolves, it is essential that adequate evaluation be undertaken to demonstrate clearly the nature of the relationship between the promise and the performance of multi-institutional systems.

REFERENCES

1. Sheldon, Alan; Barrett, Diana; and Gupta, Anil. "Managing Multi-Institutional Collaboration." Faculty Discussion Papers in Health Policy and Management, Harvard School of Public Health, March 1978.
2. *Hospitals in the 1980s: Nine Views.* Chicago: American Hospital Association, 1977.
3. Brown, Montague and Lewis, Howard L. *Hospital Management Systems: Multi-Unit Organization and Delivery of Health Care.* Germantown, MD: Aspen Systems Corporation, 1976.
4. Brown, Montague. "Multi-Institutional Arrangements: Shared Services Gain Support." *Hospitals, J.A.H.A.* 52:131-137, April 1, 1978.
5. Portnoy, Steven. "The Swelling Tide: Services and Management in Systems." *Hospitals, J.A.H.A.* 51:63-67, April 1, 1977.
6. Toomey, Robert E.; Stavros, John C.; and Sanders, Dorothy S. "Multi-Institutional Arrangements: Hospitals' Move Toward Systems Gains Momentum." *Hospitals, J.A.H.A.* 53:154-157, 192, April 1, 1979.
7. Committee on Costs of Medical Care. *Publications* 28 vols. Chicago: U. of Chicago Press, 1928-1932.
8. McNerney, Walter J. and Riedel, Donald C. *Regionalization of Rural Health Care.* Ann Arbor: The University of Michigan, 1962.
9. "Statement on Optimum Health Services." Chicago: American Hospital Association, 1965.
10. *Secretary's Advisory Committee on Hospital Effectiveness — Report.* Washington, DC, Department of Health, Education, and Welfare, October 1968.
11. P. L. 93-641, Title XV, National Health Planning and Resources Development, Part A, January 4, 1975.
12. Brown and Lewis, *Hospital Management Systems,* pp. 28-32.
13. Clark, Welden E. "The Semantics of Multihospital Aggregations." *Health Services Research.* 6:193-208, Fall 1971.
14. Starkweather, David B. "Health Facility Mergers: Some Conceptualizations." *Medical Care.* 9:468-478, November-December 1971.
15. DeVries, Robert A. "Strength in Numbers." *Hospitals, J.A.H.A.* 52:81-84, March 16, 1978.
16. Mason, Scott A. "The Multihospital Movement Defined." Paper delivered at Johns Hopkins University, Seminar Services on "The Multihospital Movement," Baltimore, MD, December 7, 1978.
17. Reynolds, James and Stunden, Ann E. "The Organization of Not-for-Profit Hospital Systems." *Health Care Management Review,* 3:23-36, Summer 1978.
18. DeVries, Robert A. "Kellogg's Role in Fostering Shared Services." *Hospitals, J.A.H.A.* 47:86-87, February 1, 1973.
19. Astolfi, Adrienne A. and Matti, Leo B. "Survey Profiles Shared Services." *Hospitals, J.A.H.A.* 46:61-65, September 16, 1972.
20. Smejda, Hellena A. "Shared Services." *Hospital Financial Management,* 5:9-15,63, March 1975.
21. Taylor, Elworth. "Participation in Shared Programs Up Sharply, Survey Discloses." *Hospitals, J.A.H.A.* 51:192, 194, 196, 198, July 16, 1977.

22. *Guidelines to Shared Services,* Health Services Research Center, Chicago, July 1971.
23. DiPaolo, Vincent. "AHS Studies Service Effectiveness." *Modern Healthcare.* 9:52, May 1979.
24. Johnson, Donald E. "30 Large Voluntary Hospitals Form National For-Profit Cooperative." *Modern Healthcare.* 7:12, November 1977.
25. Fitschen, Fred A. "Shared Services: Two Viewpoints." *Hospital and Health Services Administration.* 23:22-37, Spring 1978.
26. Danielson, John M. "Health Consortium Responds to Total Health Care Needs." *Hospitals, J.A.H.A.* 51:69-73, March 1, 1977.
27. Popoli, Alfred F. "The Quadrangle: A Working Health Consortium." *Michigan Hospitals.* 13:10-13, March 1977.
28. McDaniel, John P. "Maryland Health Care System, Inc.: A Creative Response to Change." *Health Care Management Review.* 3:29-42, Fall 1978.
29. Brown, Montague. "Contract Management: Latest Development in the Trend Towards Regionalization of Hospital and Health Services." *Hospital and Health Services Administration.* 21:40-59, Winter 1976.
30. Brown, Montague and Money, William H. "Contract Management: Is it For Your Hospital?" *Trustee.* 29:12-16, February 1976.
31. Johnson, Donald E. L. "A 29% Rise in Management Contracts Reported by Multiunit Hospital Systems." *Modern Healthcare.* 8:46-47, April 1978.
32. DiPaolo, Vincent. "Nonprofits Predict 38% Rise in Contract Business." *Modern Healthcare.* 8:47-50, April 1978.
33. Brown, Montague and Lewis, Howard L. "Small Hospitals Contract for Management Help." *Harvard Business Review.* 54:8, 13, May-June 1976.
34. Wegmiller, Donald C. "Multi-Institutional Pacts Offer Rural Hospitals Do-Or-Die Options." *Hospitals, J.A.H.A.* 52:51-54, January 16, 1978.
35. Latimer, Ben W. and Poston, Pat. "Multi-State, Multi-Service Corporate Model." *Topics in Health Care Financing.* 2:25-37, Summer 1976.
36. Downey, Gregg W. "For Sale: Hospital Management." *Modern Healthcare.* 1:35-43, June 1974.
37. Anderson, Jack R. *The Road to Recovery.* Nashville, TN: Rich Publishing Company, 1976.
38. Johnson, Donald E. L. "Jack R. Anderson: Management Firms Will Double Share of Market." *Modern Healthcare.* 7:60-62, January 1977.
39. DiPaolo, Vincent. "Rate of Contract Increases Slow." *Modern Healthcare.* 8:18-19, August 1978.
40. "Management Contract System Expected to Expand Greatly in Future Years." *Federation of American Hospitals Review.* 10:14-17, October 1977.
41. Miller, Andrew W. "Management Contracts Aid Hospitals and Bolster Growth of Companies." *Federation of American Hospitals Review.* 10:39-41, October 1977.
42. Malm, Harry M. "Multihospital Management: Analyzing An Example." *Hospital Administration.* 18:27-52, Spring 1973.
43. Brown and Lewis, *Hospital Management Systems,* pp. 148-157, 213-219, 231-237.

44. "CHA Conference Discusses Alternatives for Continuing Catholic Sponsorship of Health Care Facilities." *Modern Healthcare.* 6:21-22, June 1976.
45. "Catholic Sponsorship of Health Care Facilities." *Hospital Progress.* 58: 49-88, June 1977.
46. DiPaolo, Vincent. "Catholic Congregations Contemplate Forming a Regional Hospital Network." *Modern Healthcare.* 8:8-9, August 1978.
47. Brown and Lewis, *Hospital Management Systems*, pp. 97-103, 188-195.
48. "Prospects for Efficiencies and Economies are Leading to Creation of Multi-hospital Organizations." *Modern Hospital.* 121:39-41, July 1973.
49. Morris, Stephen M. "An Emerging Health Care System." *Hospital Administration.* 18:76-84, Spring 1973.
50. Platou, Carl N. and Rice, James A. "Multihospital Holding Companies." *Harvard Business Review.* 50:14-16, 18, 20-21, 146, 148-49, May-June 1972.
51. Platou, Carl N., et al. "The Consector Theory of Hospital Development. *Hospital Administration.* 18:61-75, Spring 1973.
52. "HCMR Interview: Carl Platou." *Health Care Management Review.* 3:87-92, Fall 1978.
53. Springate, David D. and McNeil, Melissa Craig. "Management Policies in Investor-Owned Hospitals." *Health Care Management Review.* 2:57-67, Summer 1977.
54. Baydin, Lynda Diane and Sheldon, Alan. "Corporate Models in Health Care Delivery." *Hospital Administration.* 20:40-52, Winter 1975.
55. May, J. Joel. "Economic Variables in Hospital Mergers." *Analysis of Hospital Mergers-Conference Proceedings.* Rockville, MD: National Center for Health Services Research and Development, October 1971.
56. Brown and Lewis, *Hospital Management Systems*, pp. 259-266.
57. Brown, Montague and Money, William H. "Implications of Multihospital Management for Catholic Hospitals." *Hospital Progress.* 56:89-92, September 1975.
58. Toomey, Robert E. and Toomey, Robert C. "Political Realities of Capital Formation and Capital Allocation." *Hospital and Health Services Administration.* 21:11-23, Spring 1976.
59. Malm, Harry M. "Systems Can Reduce Costs, but Need Incentives for Future Development: Lutheran Hospital and Homes Society of America." *Hospitals, J.A.H.A.* 51:63-67, March 1, 1977.
60. Hernandez, Michael D. and Howie, C. Gordon. "The Evolving Role of Multi-Hospital Systems in Health Care Financing." Paper presented at Invitational Conference on Multi-Hospital Systems and Shared Services Organizations, Washington, DC, June 15-16, 1978.
61. "Prospects for Efficiencies and Economies are Leading to Creation of Multi-hospital Organizations."
62. Tibbitts, Samuel J. "Multiple Hospital Systems." *Hospital Administration.* 18:10-20, Spring 1973.
63. Brown and Lewis, *Hospital Management Systems*, p. 266.
64. Toomey, Robert E. "The Strength of Systems." *Hospital Progress.* 59:52-56, November 1978.

65. Wegmiller, Donald C. "From a Hospital to a Health Care System: A Case Example." *Health Care Management Review.* 3:61-67, Winter 1978.
66. McCool, Barbara P. "Management of Human Resources in Collaborative Arrangements." *Topics in Health Care Financing.* 2:51-58, Summer 1976.
67. Westerman, John H. "Quality of Care as Addressed Through Corporate Arrangements." Paper presented at Invitational Conference on Multi-Hospital Systems and Shared Services Organizations, Washington, DC, June 15-16, 1978.
68. Brown, Montague. "Multiple-Unit Hospital Systems Under Single Management." *Hospital and Health Services Administration.* 21:88-95, Spring 1976.
69. "HCMR Interview: Carl Platou."
70. Johnson, "Jack R. Anderson . . . "
71. Latimer, Ben W. "Systems That Secure Resources Help Ensure Hospitals' Survival." *Hospitals, J.A.H.A.* 51:57-58, 60-61, March 1, 1977.
72. McCool, "Management of Human Resources . . . "
73. Brown, Montague. "The Promise of Multihospital Management." *Hospital Progress.* 56:36-42, August 1975.
74. Milburn, Jack. "Shared Management Expertise Spells Survival for the Small." *Hospitals, J.A.H.A.* 50:52-54, February 1976.
75. Friedrich, Paul and Ross, Austin. "Consortium Serves Rural Hospitals' Educational Needs." *Hospitals, J.A.H.A.* 51:95-96, March 1, 1977.
76. Rapaport, Gary D. "Critical Look at the Motives for Hospital Mergers." *Hospital Forum.* 18:9-12, June 1975.
77. Wegmiller, "Multi-Institutional Pacts . . . "
78. "Catholic Sponsorship . . . "
79. Toomey, "The Strength of Systems."
80. Brown and Lewis, *Hospital Management Systems*, pp. 266-271.
81. *Services Shared By Health Care Organizations*, Volumes 1-4. Health Services Research Center of the Hospital Research and Educational Trust and Northwestern University, Chicago, May 1977.
82. Biggs, Errol L. "Accountability in Corporation Managed and Traditionally Managed Nonprofit Hospitals." Ph.D. dissertation, The Pennsylvania State University, 1977.
83. DiPaolo, Vincent. "Bills Are Lower in Contracted Units." *Modern Healthcare.* 8:13-14, January 1978.
84. Treat, Thomas F. "The Performance of Merging Hospitals." *Medical Care.* 14:199-209, March 1976.
85. Neumann, Bruce R. "Financial Analysis of a Hospital Merger: Samaritan Health Service." *Medical Care.* 12:983-998, December 1974.
86. Edwards, Sam A. *Demonstration and Evaluation of Integrated Health Care Facilities, Samaritan Health Service; Phoenix, Arizona*, Volumes I-IV, Health Services Research Center of the Hospital Research and Educational Trust and Northwestern University, Chicago, June 1972.
87. Edwards, Sam A. and Astolfi, Adrienne A. "Merger: Cause and Effect." *Hospital Administration.* 18:24-33, Summer 1973.

88. Edwards, Sam A. and Astolfi, Adrienne A. "Study Analyzes Effects of Delivery of Health Services Through a Multihospital System." *Hospitals, J.A.H.A.* 47:44-49, February 16, 1973.

89. Cooney, James P., Jr., and Alexander, Thomas L. *Multihospital Systems: An Evaluation*, Parts One - Four. Health Services Research Center of the Hospital Research and Educational Trust and Northwestern University, Chicago, 1975.

90. Cooney and Alexander, *Multihospital Systems: An Evaluation.*

91. Alexander, Thomas; Money, William; and Beatzoglou, Tryfon. "Multihospital Systems May Offer Solutions to Delivery Problems." *Hospitals, J.A.H.A.* 50:73-76, November 1, 1976.

92. "Multihospital Systems: The Older They Get, the Better They Run." *Trustee.* 29:32-33, December 1976.

93. Coyne, Joseph S. "A Comparative Study of the Performance and Characteristics of Multihospital Systems." Ph.D. dissertation, The University of California, Berkeley, 1978.

94. Treat, "The Performance of Merging Hospitals."

95. Cooney and Alexander, *Multihospital Systems: An Evaluation.*

96. Edwards, *Demonstration and Evaluation of Integrated. . .*

97. Cooney and Alexander, *Multihospital Systems: An Evaluation.*

98. Edwards and Astolfi, "Merger: Cause and Effect."

99. Edwards and Astolfi, "Study Analyzes Effects . . . "

100. Alexander, Money, and Beatzoglou, "Multihospital Systems May Offer . . ."

101. "Multihospital Systems: The Older They Get . . . "

102. *Services Shared by Health Organizations.*

103. Biggs, "Accountability in Corporation Managed . . . "

104. Treat, "The Performance of Merging Hospitals."

105. Edwards, *Demonstration and Evaluation of Integrated . . .*

106. Neumann, "Financial Analysis of a Hospital Merger . . . "

107. Cooney and Alexander, *Multihospital Systems: An Evaluation.*

108. Cooney and Alexander, *Multihospital Systems: An Evaluation.*

109. Brown, Montague. "Multi-hospital Systems and Shared Services: Some Questions and Issues." Paper presented at the Invitational Conference on Multi-Hospital Systems and Shared Services, Washington, DC, June 15-16, 1978.

110. *Regionalization of Patient Care: Case Studies of Interhospital Sharing*, Volumes 1-4. Silver Springs, MD: Macro Systems, Inc., October 1976.

111. Starkweather, David B. "Is Big Beautiful?" Paper delivered at Annual Meeting of Association of University Programs in Health Administration, Chicago, May 8, 1978.

112. Studnicki, James. "Multihospital Systems: A Research Perspective." Paper presented at Johns Hopkins University, Seminar Series on "The Multihospital Movement," Baltimore, MD, December 14, 1978.

113. Vraciu, Robert A. and Zuckerman, Howard S. "Legal and Financial Constraints on the Development and Growth of Multiple Hospital Arrangements." *Health Care Management Review.* 4:39-47, Winter 1979.

114. Starkweather, David B.; Greenawalt, Leo; and Mehringer, Anne. *Anti-Trust Implications of Hospital Mergers: A Review and Discussion.* Health Policy Monograph Series, Blue Cross-Blue Shield Association, June 1979.
115. Starkweather, "Is Big Beautiful?"
116. Cooney and Alexander. *Multihospital Systems: An Evaluation.*
117. Starkweather, Greenawalt, and Mehringer. *Anti-Trust Implications . . .*
118. Horty, John F. "Court Ruling Could Outlaw Joint Hospital Efforts to Cut Rising Costs." *Modern Healthcare.* 6:58, 62, August 1976.
119. Borsody, Robert P. "Hospitals Enter Antitrust Era." *Hospitals, J.A.H.A.* 52:59-63, May 1, 1978.
120. "Congress Sidesteps Antitrust Issue." *Modern Healthcare.* 9:19, May 1979.
121. "Agency Regulatory Actions Do Not Violate Antitrust Laws, U.S. District Court Says." *Hospital Week.* 15:2, March 23, 1979.
122. Vraciu and Zuckerman, "Legal and Financial Constraints . . . "
123. Bromberg, Robert S. "Tax Considerations in Forming Shared Services Organizations." *Hospitals, J.A.H.A.* 51:49-56, March 1, 1977.
124. Bromberg, Robert S. "The Conflict Between Tax Policy and Cost Containment." *Trustee.* 30:8-11, August 1977.
125. Vraciu and Zuckerman, "Legal and Financial Constraints . . . "
126. Horty, John F. "Court Says IRS Can't Tax Shared Laundry." *Modern Healthcare.* 8:72, 74, September 1978.
127. Vraciu and Zuckerman, "Legal and Financial Constraints . . . "
128. Reifsnyder, Edward F. "The Financial Impact of Regulation and Legislation on Multi-Hospital Systems and Shared Services Organizations." Paper presented at the Invitational Conference on Multi-Hospital Systems and Shared Services Organizations, Washington, DC, June 15-16, 1978.
129. "Toomey Charges Medicare Discriminates Against Nonprofits." *Hospital Progress.* 59:23, October 1978.
130. Diamond, Alvin D. "Health Financing: Multi-Hospital Systems and Shared Service Organizations." Paper presented at the Invitational Conference on Multi-Hospital Systems and Shared Services Organizations, Washington, DC, June 15-16, 1978.
131. Toomey and Toomey, "Political Realities of Capital . . . "
132. "Regulations Discouraging Chains, Shared Services." *Modern Healthcare.* 8:9-10, August 1978.
133. Lang, Wendy. "Reimbursement to Multihospital Systems." Master's thesis, The University of Michigan, Program in Hospital Administration, 1977.
134. Bromberg, "Tax Considerations in Forming . . . "
135. Vraciu and Zuckerman, "Legal and Financial Constraints . . . "
136. "Regulations Discouraging Chains . . . "
137. Wegmiller, Donald C. "Legislation and Regulation: Impact On and Opportunities for Multi-Hospital Systems and Shared Service Organizations." Paper presented at the Invitational Conference on Multi-Hospital Systems and Shared Services Organizations, Washington, DC, June 15-16, 1978.
138. Wegmiller, "Legislation and Regulation . . . "

139. "Self-insured Chains Show Big Savings." *Modern Healthcare*. 7:17-18, October 1977.
140. Lang, "Reimbursement to Multihospital Systems."
141. Diamond, "Health Financing . . . "
142. Enright, Michael. "Competition, Cooperation and Sharing." *Topics in Health Care Financing*. 2:99-108, Summer 1976.
143. Johnson, George O. and Litman, Theodore J. "Management of Shared Services." *Topics in Health Care Financing-Shared Services*. 2:87-97, Summer 1976.
144. McDaniel, "Maryland Health Care System . . . "
145. Danielson, "Health Consortium Responds . . . "
146. Brown and Money, "Contract Management . . . "
147. Latimer, Ben W. "Developing Multihospital Arrangements: Some Practical Considerations." *Hospital Progress*. 57:62-67, October 1976.
148. Platou and Rice, "Multihospital Holding Companies."
149. Rothman, Robert A.; Schwartzbaum, Arthur M.; and McCarthy, John H. "Physicians and a Hospital Merger: Patterns of Resistance to Organizational Change." *Journal of Health and Social Behavior*. 12:46-55, March 1971.
150. Rourke, Anthony J. J. "Mergers: The Physician's Concern." *The Hospital Medical Staff*. 1:19-24, October 19729 1:17-20, November 1972; 1:31-35, December 1972.
151. Downey, "For Sale: Hospital Management."
152. Cooney and Alexander, *Multihospital Systems: An Evaluation.*
153. Blumberg, Arthur and Wiener, William. "One from Two: Facilitating an Organizational Merger." *Journal of Applied Behavioral Science*. 7:87-102, January - February 1971.
154. Wortman, Paul M. "Merger Implementation: An Organizational Evaluation." Technical report, Northwestern University, undated.
155. Johnson and Litman, "Management of Shared Services."
156. Crews, James C. "Human Concerns About Hospital Mergers." *Hospitals, J.A.H.A.* 48:79-83, June 1974.
157. Starkweather, David B. "Beyond the Semantics of Multihospital Aggregations." *Health Service Research*. 7:58-61, Spring 1972.
158. MacStravic, Robin E. "Multi-Hospital Systems: Vertical Integration." Paper delivered at Invitational Conference on Multi-Hospital Systems and Shared Services Organizations, Washington, DC, June 15-16, 1978.
159. Starkweather, "Health Facility Mergers . . . "
160. Toomey, Robert E. "Community vs. Specialized Medicine." *Hospitals, J.A.H.A.* 45:43-46, May 16, 1971.
161. Connors, Edward J. "Generic Problems in the Development and Operation of Multihospital Systems." Paper delivered at the Sixth Annual Conference on Multihospital Systems, San Francisco, July 17-19, 1978.
162. Farley, James T. "The Multi-Hospital Challenge." *Michigan Hospitals*. 14:26-27, October 1978.
163. Toomey, Robert E. "County Facilities Equitably Serve All Residents: Greenville (SC) Hospital System." *Hospitals, J.A.H.A.* 51:75-76, 78, March 1, 1977.

164. "HCMR Interview: Bob Toomey." *Health Care Management Review.* 2:77-86, Summer 1977.
165. Sigmond, Robert M. "The Issues Facing Multihospital Systems." Paper delivered at the Sixth Annual Conference on Multihospital Systems, San Francisco, July 17-19, 1978.
166. Stull, Richard J. "Many Concepts Mold Multi-institutional Systems." *Hospitals, J.A.H.A.* 51:43-45, March 1, 1977.
167. Levitan, Mark. "The Core Teaching Hospital and Multi-Hospital Systems." Paper delivered at the Multi-Hospital Systems/University Teaching Hospitals Conference, Chicago, August 21-22, 1978.
168. "Merging Teaching Hospitals, Multihospital Systems Eyed." *Hospitals, J.A.H.A.* 52:21-22, September 16, 1978.
169. Wegmiller, Donald C. "Implications of Multihospital System Development for University/Teaching Hospitals." Paper presented at the Multi-Hospital Systems/University Teaching Hospitals Conference, Chicago, August 21-22, 1978.
170. Wegmiller, "Implications of Multihospital . . . "
171. Warden, Gail L. and Sinioris, Marie E. "Medical School Based Sharing." *Topics in Health Care Financing.* 2:39-49, Summer 1976.
172. Campbell, James A. and Sinioris, Marie E. "Shoulder to Shoulder: A Role of a University Teaching Hospital in a Multihospital System: A Case Study of the Rush University System for Health." Paper presented at the Multi-Hospital Systems/University Teaching Hospitals Conference, Chicago, August 21-22, 1978.
173. Lowe, John M. "Program Notes." W. K. Kellogg Foundation, January 19, 1979.
174. Arnwine, Don L. "Multihospital System Implications." Paper presented at the Multi-Hospital Systems/University Teaching Hospitals Conference, Chicago, August 21-22, 1978.
175. Warden, Gail L. "A Rationale for a New Relationship Between Multi-Hospital Systems and Teaching Hospitals." Paper presented at the Multi-Hospital Systems/University Teaching Hospitals Conference, Chicago, August 21-22, 1978.
176. Ross, Austin. "Vertically Linked Organizations Hold Challenges–and Opportunities." *Hospitals, J.A.H.A.* 53:67-72, January 16, 1979.
177. "HCMR Interview: Carl Platou."
178. Brown and Lewis, *Hospital Management Systems*, pp. 259-260.
179. Johnson and Litman, "Management of Shared Services."
180. Sheldon, Alan and Barrett, Diana. "The Janus Principle." *Health Care Management Review.* 2:77-87, Spring 1977.
181. Sheldon, Barrett, and Gupta, "Managing Multi-Institutional Collaboration."
182. Brown, Montague. "Changing Role of the Administrator in Multiple Hospital Systems." *Hospital and Health Services Administration.* 23:6-19, Fall 1978.
183. Shortell, Stephen. "Managerial Models." *Hospital Progress.* 58:64-68, October 1977.

184. Johnson, Donald E. L. "Continuing Education Programs for Hospital Managers Expanding Rapidly." *Modern Healthcare.* 8:40-44, December 1978.
185. Coyne, "A Comparative Study . . . "
186. Prybil, Lawrence and Starkweather, David B. "Current Perspectives on Hospital Governance." *Hospital and Health Services Administration.* 21:67-75, Fall 1976.
187. Porter, Karen W. "Think System, Not Institution, Hospital Trustees Told." *Trustee.* 31:41-43, February 1978.
188. Shortell, "Managerial Models."
189. Connors, Edward J. and Miriam, Sr. Christa. "Catholic Hospital System Responds to View of Future." *Hospitals, J.A.H.A.* 51:79-81, March 1, 1977.
190. Burns, Sr. Elizabeth Mary. "Developing a Catholic Health Care System." *Hospital Progress.* 57:48-54, 80, December 1976.
191. Schweiker, Hon. Richard S. "Multi-Institutional Arrangements from a Political Perspective." Paper delivered at the Invitational Conference on Multi-Hospital Systems and Shared Services Organizations, Washington, DC, June 15-16, 1978.
192. Starkweather, "Is Big Beautiful?"

Part II

Case
Descriptions

Introduction

In this section, to be presented are descriptions of 10 selected multi-institutional systems. In each instance, the system has been the recipient of grant funding from the W. K. Kellogg Foundation which has served as "seed money" for further growth and development. The types of institutional relationships to be discussed are primarily shared services, management contracts, and lease arrangements. As will be seen, several different organizational models have been employed by the systems in establishing their networks.

The primary source of information was material made available from the Kellogg Foundation files, including grant proposals, progress reports, and field observations. These were supplemented by journal articles, communication with key personnel in the systems, and, in three cases, visits to the sites. The descriptions have been organized to first provide background information on the purpose for which the arrangements were created, the problems to be addressed, and the objectives sought. Then described for each system is the structure of the organization, followed by the process of operation, including organizational strategies.

Case descriptions in this section were written by David P. Smith, Kathryn Walker, and Howard S. Zuckerman. At the time of the writing, Mr. Smith and Ms. Walker were graduate students in the Program in Hospital Administration at The University of Michigan.

Finally, the outcome resulting from the systems' activities is discussed. Data limitations and, in several instances, the relatively recent development of the systems, constrain the degree to which assessment of the outcome can be made. However, to the extent feasible, the impact of these 10 systems is considered in terms of economic, manpower, and organizational benefits achieved.

Billings Deaconess Hospital–
Montana-Wyoming Health Resources

Background and Structure

Montana-Wyoming Health Resources (MWHR), an operating division of Billings Deaconess Hospital, represents an attempt to develop vertical integration of health care delivery through the vehicle of management services contracts. The MWHR effort resulted from a broadened view of the future role of the hospital and a recognition of the problems of many nonhospital organizations involved in meeting community health needs. The words of its originators serve to explain:

> . . . the role of the hospital in the delivery of health care services is undergoing a transition and redefinition. Witness the expansion of hospitals into non-acute care functions and programs such as neighborhood health centers, nursing homes, health maintenance organizations . . . and other unique service delivery concepts. (The hospital administrator's) purview must extend beyond the acute care institution . . . Hospitals, as the major and most differentiated unit in the health care system, must direct efforts at integrating the components of care with regard to prevention, early detection, acute care, and rehabilitation/aftercare.
>
> The problems faced by hospitals . . . are not unique to the hospital industry. There are thousands of nonhospital health care agencies providing an array of services directly concerned with the health and welfare of citizens in their communities. Their management problems and financial plight are similar to those faced in the

hospital. The same constraints face them–public demands for accountability, manpower problems, federal regulation, financing, and lack of management expertise.[1]

Billings Deaconess saw the fulfillment of this vision and solution to the problems to be a function of a variety of parameters, among the most important being the management function. Management services contracts were seen as an appropriate vehicle by which management skills could be improved and access to management support services be realized.[2] A study of the market in eastern Montana and northern Wyoming, done in 1975 by the firm of Peat, Marwick, Mitchell, and Company, concluded that most of the elements for a comprehensive, cooperative health care system in the region were then available and that Deaconess should proceed in the development of a program to coordinate the sharing of resources among the various health care institutions and health-related agencies.[3]

Deaconess identified seven program objectives to guide the development of the system:[4]

1. To develop a network of resources for care whose operations are closely coordinated and designed to make each necessary service as accessible as possible to the population of all parts of the service area.
2. To develop a manner, style, and setting to meet with dignity and understanding the health care needs of people in the region, and to assist in establishing a setting in which the health care providers can render a needed service in a professional and satisfying manner.
3. To provide for health services in a manner consistent with recognized standards emphasizing effectiveness and efficiency.
4. To provide the personnel necessary for all levels of care and/or service in the health care system.
5. To develop and maintain relationships and mechanisms necessary to ensure coordinated, effective, efficient, high quality care while allowing for various approaches to the delivery of services.
6. To assure that funding mechanisms provide incentives for effective, efficient, high quality care at the lowest possible cost.
7. To teach the consumer about personal health care and resources in order to have a sharing with the provider of their mutual responsibility for maintaining the consumer's health.

Vertical integration through management services contracts began in 1975 when Deaconess reached agreements with two nonhospital providers: the Rimrock Guidance Foundation and the South Central Montana Regional Mental Health Center.

The Rimrock Guidance Foundation is a multiservice chemical dependency counseling, education, and treatment agency. The agreement between the Foundation and Deaconess most closely approaches the traditional management contract model. Deaconess provides a full-time Executive Director to the Foundation along with several management support services including accounting, data processing, educational services, planning, and personnel management.[5]

The agreement with the Mental Health Center is more complex, representing an attempt to address vertical integration in the areas of clinical services, policy making, facilities, and staff.[6] The Center is a comprehensive mental health agency providing services to 11 counties via 10 satellite offices. The contract calls for Deaconess to provide a full-time administrative officer, chosen with the advice and consent of the Center's governing board, to serve as Deputy Director of the Center. The Center retains its own Director, who is a psychiatrist. Billings Deaconess provides management support services and consultation to the Center in the areas of finance, personnel management, purchasing, and other services as necessary to meet Center objectives. The Center reimburses Deaconess for the Deputy Director's salary, fringe benefits, and related expenses, while the general management support services are billed at a prearranged hourly rate varying with the level of hospital personnel involved in providing the service, all subject to a limit on the total sum to be paid for the year. Deaconess also provides the Center with data processing services, primarily in the areas of programming for patient billing and utilization monitoring. Certain of the day-to-day data processing functions are performed by an employee provided by Deaconess. Payment for this service is based on the lower of audited expenses or a prearranged fee schedule. General maintenance and housekeeping services are also provided and billed according to expenses incurred.[7]

In return, the Center uses the 21 bed inpatient psychiatric services of Deaconess as part of its comprehensive mental health program. Deaconess is responsible for providing nursing services and other customary patient support functions while the Center remains responsible for the clinical evaluation, treatment, and rehabilitation of the patients. The Center Director and contracted community psychiatrists hold joint appointments on both the Center and Deaconess medical staffs. The Center is responsible for the in-service training and consultation services needed by Deaconess' nursing and ancillary department staffs in relation to their duties in caring for Center patients.[8]

As part of the agreement, Deaconess and the Center combine in the joint provision of group home services for deinstitutionalized patients. Deaconess provides the facilities and certain basic services, such as food and maintenance, while the Center is responsible for patient management and overall administration of facility operations. The Center reimburses Deaconess on a per patient per diem basis.[9]

These arrangements are all part of a one year contract, subject to annual renewal. Either party may request a review of the contract terms at any time and the parties may agree to revise any or all terms at a mutually agreeable time. The contract is subject to termination upon 90 day written notice. All Deaconess employees involved remain responsible to Deaconess Hospital, which acts as an independent contractor in the performance of its duties.[10]

Support for vertical integration as a means to provide high quality patient care and service continuity is felt by Deaconess to begin at the board policy making level. A committee of the Deaconess governing board was established in 1976 to study their hospital's role and to make recommendations regarding the integration of services into a comprehensive system of care. Several board members from Deaconess hold joint appointments to the governing board of the Rimrock Guidance Foundation, indicating just one example of policy level integration among the affiliated institutions.[11]

In 1977, Deaconess approached the W. K. Kellogg Foundation with a request for grant funding to support more rapid development of the contract services program. The Kellogg Foundation offered assistance amounting to $173,260 on a declining basis over a three year period to cover the costs of salaries for new staff, travel, education, marketing, and outside consulting services. This amount was to be supplemented by anticipated service revenues of the program amounting to $772,900. A target of five new management contracts on multiple-shared-services contracts within the three year period was established. The program was expected to be self-supporting by the end of the third year.[12]

Deaconess determined that an organizational vehicle with an identity separate from, but related to, the Billings Deaconess Hospital would be the most appropriate means by which to pursue the management services program. "Political implications" were identified as the reason behind this decision: small rural hospitals were seen as sensitive about maintaining their autonomy from Deaconess while larger competing hospitals in

Billings had expressed concern over changes in patient referral patterns that might result from affiliations between the small rural hospitals and Deaconess.[13] Thus, Montana-Wyoming Health Resources was born, standing as an operating division of the Deaconess Hospital and sharing the same 501 (c) (3) status assigned to Deaconess.

Implementation and Process

Other than some penetration by the Lutheran Hospital and Homes Society and several Catholic orders, Deaconess viewed the multi-unit health care delivery market in eastern Montana and northern Wyoming to be essentially untapped. Consistent with their interest in vertical integration, MWHR saw their potential market to consist of any organization providing health care or health care related services, such as rehabilitation programs, public education and referral agencies, handicapped service centers, counseling programs, or county nursing agencies.[14] In the first year of the grant period, MWHR staff visited 13 target hospitals to inform the administrators of the objectives of the program and the services available. Similar meetings were held with the Montana Hospital Association, the Montana Health Systems Agency, the Director of Montana Social and Rehabilitative Services, the District Learning Center, the Director of Regional Medical Education of the University of Montana, and various city and county health departments. Such meetings served not only as informative sessions but also assisted MWHR in determining the perceived priority needs of these organizations around which services could be designed.

This tactic was part of an overall marketing strategy designed to approach management contracts incrementally. The strategy and its rationale are explained in a MWHR report:

> The political issues and concerns of the target institutions . . . make it inadvisable to make a proposal for . . . comprehensive contract management as an initial step . . . In most cases it appears necessary to demonstrate a mutual concern for the viability and autonomy of the target institutions by way of general shared services offerings before there is a chance of having a comprehensive management contract accepted. For this reason, some specific shared services programs were developed around the identified priority needs of the regions and the available resources with which to serve those needs.[15]

MWHR also believes that, in attempting to secure management contracts, a concerted effort should be made to develop a rapport with governing boards and medical staff, as well as administrators, of target institutions. Only then, they believe, is it reasonable to propose a comprehensive management contract.[16]

Several priority needs were identified by this process:[17]

1. Professional recruiting and professional education
2. Group purchasing
3. Computerized data processing
4. Financial management

MWHR then sought to develop specific shared services in these areas to be made available on a selective or "unbundled" basis rather than as a set of services that can be purchased only as a package.

To address some of the needs in the area of professional manpower, a Health Professions Registry is being developed. The Registry will provide back-up support to affiliating institutions attempting to meet manpower shortages as a result of vacations, resignations, and leaves. The Registry will also attempt to arrange for the sharing of contracted professional personnel such as physical therapists, the employment cost for which would be prohibitive for single institutions. Professional and consumer education programs have begun with nursing seminars in coronary care and infection control, and a consumer education course on medical care in the home.

The group purchasing program represents an example of MWHR's determination to enlist the support of outside assistance where their own expertise or resources are not sufficient to provide certain services. It also provides an example of cooperation between multi-unit systems. In this case it was determined that a broad based group purchasing program was beyond the scope of local resources. Health Central, Inc., a nonprofit multi-unit organization with corporate offices in Minneapolis, with a large group purchasing program, was contracted with to provide this service. MWHR has also used Health Central in a variety of other consultative roles such as data processing consultations for both Deaconess Hospital and the Regional Mental Health Center and for assistance with biomedical engineering services provided by MWHR.[18] This latter service provides for electrical and biomedical equipment surveys, including on-site inspection of all electrically sensitive patient areas and patient care equipment.

Financial management contracts were established with the Rimrock Foundation, and two small rural hospitals in Montana in 1978. The financial management package includes accounting services, budget development, cash flow planning, cost reports, systems design, and rate review assistance.

A regional computerized ECG analysis service represents one more contracted service available to affiliates. Nine hospitals had signed on for this service as of 1977. MWHR also offers computerized data processing through the Deaconess computer, as illustrated earlier in the agreement with the Regional Mental Health Center.

The bulk of the responsibility for coordination and implementation of the program is assigned to a project director. He serves as the contact person with the administration and governing board of contracting institutions. He assists in coordinating the services of consultants and technical staff in precontract assessments, aiding administrators of contracting institutions, and in preparing information sessions to be conducted for board members, administrators, and other community groups. Two accountants with special expertise in health care finance were hired to provide financial management services.

Impact and Outcome

The short time since the project began and the limited data available make it difficult to provide substantial assessment of the program thus far. Evaluation protocols are, however, being developed by MWHR to assess the impact of the program and these will be used to direct future activities. The Health Professions Registry, financial management services, data processing, biomedical engineering, and computerized ECG programs, to the extent that they are well designed and properly implemented, have obvious implications for improving the quantity and quality of services and financial status of the participants. For instance, precontract audits performed for the group purchasing program have indicated potential savings of approximately 20 percent.[19] The group home services detailed earlier was a direct result of previous service agreements between Deaconess and the Regional Mental Health Center and offers evidence of the potential of the MWHR program to act as a catalyst in the development of new clinical and therapeutic services in its service area.

In early 1979, MWHR entered into another management contract, bringing the total of managed organizations to three. Consistent with the goal of vertical integration, the new contract is with the McCone County Hospital and Nursing Home in Circle, Montana. The 20 bed hospital and 40 bed nursing home were previously separate organizations, now combined under one board and one management. MWHR is also being considered by four other health care institutions for management contracts.[20] These two reports testify to slow but steady progress in introducing the management contract model to the MWHR service area.

MWHR itself sees its main contribution to date to be in the establishment of the groundwork for cooperation upon which the promise of such cooperation can be tested. They report that:

> ... our experience indicates that the benefits derived are much greater than the revenue derived. A dialogue is established among the managers of the agencies, and a problem solving forum is developed. With the autonomy of each organization remaining intact, the employees are able to communicate about referral and service delivery problems. The personnel which are shared among several users gain an insight into the problems of managing community health services. Organizational barriers to service integration, though not entirely removed, are diminished.[21]

REFERENCES

1. Billings Deaconess Hospital, "Contract Management Service Proposal for Eastern Montana and Northern Wyoming," presented to the W. K. Kellogg Foundation, May 1977.
2. Ibid.
3. Billings Deaconess Hospital, "Progress Report—A Billings Deaconess Hospital Contract Management Grant Project," submitted to the W.K. Kellogg Foundation, Winter 1978.
4. Billings Deaconess Hospital, "Contract Management Service Proposal for Eastern Montana and Northern Wyoming . . . "
5. Ibid.
6. Ibid.
7. "Agreement Between South Central Montana Regional Mental Health Center and Billings Deaconess Hospital," January 1977.
8. Ibid.
9. Ibid.
10. Ibid.
11. Billings Deaconess Hospital, "Contract Management Service Proposal for Eastern Montana and Northern Wyoming . . . "
12. DeVries, Robert A. *Program Notes:* W. K. Kellogg Foundation, June 16, 1977.
13. Billings Deaconess Hospital, "First Year Annual Report," submitted to the W. K. Kellogg Foundation, August 1978.
14. Billings Deaconess Hospital, "Contract Management Service Proposal for Eastern Montana and Northern Wyoming . . . "
15. Billings Deaconess Hospital, "First Year Annual Report . . . "
16. Billings Deaconess Hospital, "Progress Report—Billings Deaconess Hospital Contract Management Grant Project . . . "
17. Ibid.
18. Ibid.
19. Billings Deaconess Hospital, "First Year Annual Report . . . "
20. Telephone conversation with Gene O'Hara, Project Director, March 8, 1979.
21. Danielson, Donald. "Vertical Integration of Health Care Services Through Management Support Services Contracts," *The Eclectic*, The University of Michigan Program in Hospital Administration Alumni Association, Winter 1979.

Carolinas Hospital and Health Services, Inc.

Background and Structure

Carolinas Hospital and Health Services, Inc. (CHHS) was founded by the state hospital associations of North and South Carolina in 1969. CHHS is a freestanding, nonprofit, shared services corporation, organized into divisions representing the following separate but related functional shared services:

1. Carolinas Hospital Improvement Program (CHIP) provides management engineering services.
2. Carolinas Hospital Engineering Support Services (CHESS) provides plant, clinical engineering and biomedical instrumentation services.
3. Carolinas Affiliated Purchasing Program (CAPP).
4. Medical Claims Collection Bureau (MCCB).
5. Facilities Development Services (FDS) provides various services related to the management of renovation and new construction projects.
6. SIGMA, a taxpaying division providing various CHHS services to organizations not regularly served by other divisions, primarily outside of North and South Carolina.
7. CHHS Management Services (CHHS/MS) provides comprehensive management contract services.

The distinctive relationship between CHHS and the two hospital associations is characterized by CHHS President Ben W. Latimer in the following way:

> Though independent of direct association control or ownership, CHHS does serve *in effect* [emphasis in original] as the association's operational arm for some services developed or wanted by them for hospital members . . . However, CHHS is not limited to direct association initiative in service development and may operate as an expansion-minded company would in assessing user needs and organizing services to meet them.[1]

Overall governing authority rests with a board of trustees, combining broad based representation from medicine, hospital administrators and trustees, civic leaders, and the academic community. Hospital association direction is evidenced by the direct selection of 8 of 18 trustees, 2 of whom are the Associations' chief executives.[2]

The shared services approach, involving the coordinated or otherwise explicitly agreed upon sharing of responsibility for the provision of medical or nonmedical services on the part of two or more otherwise independent health care institutions, has been viewed as a means by which to meet the need for greater capability within the field. In rural areas the need is acute, but the capacity to develop such a response is limited because of an insufficient "critical mass" of volume and resources.[3] It was the recognition of such a situation in the Carolinas that led to the initial development of CHHS as an organization devoted solely to the provision of shared services.

CHHS's first services were in special need and technical management areas such as management engineering, group purchasing, and clinical engineering. It soon became apparent, however, that the regulatory, technological, and professional imperatives impinging upon small rural hospitals necessitated a more substantial response in terms of enhanced capability in many areas of management. Experience in marketing three functional shared services revealed the earliest, most successful, and most enthusiastic users were hospitals already possessing a fairly high degree of management capability. Where management depth was lacking, there was a concomitant inability to define the needs or to use the functional services effectively.[4] What existed was a management gap: a need for management depth but insufficient resources, financial or otherwise, to attract a high level manager or a specialized administrative staff. It was from this dilemma that arose Comprehensive Management Services Division of CHHS, a sophisticated, centralized, corporate management team serving a number of hospitals on a contractual basis.

The CHHS/MS program is best described as a full management-without-ownership model. CHHS/MS and the participating hospital contract with each other whereby, for a fee, CHHS/MS agrees to provide complete management of the institution while the hospital governing board retains ownership control and all legal rights and responsibilities. Under this agreement, CHHS/MS recruits and provides the hospital with an inhospital director (administrator), who has a dual reporting responsibility, reporting to both the local hospital board and to a CHHS Area Director. Area Directors, in turn, report to the CHHS Vice President for Management Services. The inhospital director performs the same duties as an administrator in a conventional setting, but relies on the back-up of CHHS/MS core staff specialists operating out of the central corporate headquarters for specialized assistance in the areas of financial management, management engineering, plant and clinical engineering, communications, and overall development coordination. The management services package involves participation in the CAPP purchasing program and, at separate cost, the optional use of CHHS's data processing services. As another option—now more often the rule than the exception—CHHS may provide the services of a chief financial officer as part of the contract package. As with the inhospital director, the chief financial officer is employed by CHHS but assigned full time to the hospital, reporting to the inhospital director.

CHHS invests no money in the hospitals and has no proprietary control over hospital earnings. CHHS's role is thus limited to one of service as opposed to a source of capital. It should be noted, however, that a recent self-evaluation study at CHHS concluded that the system ". . . should not be limited to contract management but should retain the flexibility to enter into at-risk models for hospital operations, with leasing given consideration before purchase."[5]

Remuneration for management contract services is in the form of an annual fee paid by the hospital. Early practice called for a flat rate fee. As the program evolved, the fee became a percentage of adjusted gross patient revenue (adjustments for contractual allowances and a deduction for bad debts and charity care). The percentage of revenues basis is felt to offer an incentive to CHHS to improve occupancy and operating efficiencies, in addition to being seen as an equitable way to achieve "fair share" fees among participating hospitals without constantly renegotiating contract terms.[6] The fee includes the inhospital director's salary. CHHS intends to remain flexible in its fee mechanism to adjust to the circumstances of each potential client hospital. They believe their fees to be substantially below those charged by investor-owned chains, yet offering equivalent services in the same geographic area.[7]

CHHS expects several advantages to accrue from the full management-without-ownership model. Two aspects are of particular interest: the maintenance of local board control and autonomy, and the ability to attract and apply relatively sophisticated management expertise to small rural hospitals.

It is felt that one barrier preventing the small hospital from becoming involved in multi-unit arrangements via the various lease, merger, subsidiary, kingpin, and chain models has been a fear of loss of control, divided loyalties, and institutional neglect. Local civic pride is also important in this regard. By featuring local board autonomy and control, these fears should be lessened or overcome. This feature should also help to preempt opposition from the medical staff. CHHS's status as a non-provider and hence a noncompetitor may be advantageous in overcoming these fears as well. At the same time, maintaining a local board with real power helps to identify the hospital as a community enterprise. This should be of benefit in influencing the politics of local financing and regional planning.[8] Acknowledging the sensitivities of local control, contracts have generally been for an initial term of one year. The contracts are automatically renewed unless 90 day notice is given by either party of intent to terminate or modify the contract. CHHS is presently considering lengthening the contract period given that front-end implementation costs are considerable and that the results of the contract are more visible after the first year.[9]

In an attempt to guide itself and the local governing boards it serves, and to establish general criteria against which operations can be judged, CHHS/MS explicitly set forth a set of goals, principles, and purposes.[10] Divided into guidelines for system operation and hospital operation, they are presented here to best indicate the scope and framework of the CHHS/MS model as they see it.[11]

CHHS/MS Goals for System Operation

The overall purpose of the Management Services Division of Carolinas Hospital and Health Services, Inc. is to assist and improve the voluntary health system so that the health needs of the citizenry are better met, by providing economical and community-controlled management for health care facilities. CHHS/MS will endeavor to carry out this broad purpose by working toward the following goals:

1. To benefit hospitals . . .
2. To fit comprehensive services to the needs of hospitals . . .

3. To provide reasonable service agreements that clearly detail components of service . . .
4. To assure local control . . .
5. To provide service at economical costs . . .
6. To involve community and hospital representatives in service developments . . .

CHHS/MS Goals for Hospital Operation

CHHS/MS management activity within the hospital will be directed toward the following broad goals:

1. To enable the hospital to meet the perceived health care needs of the community, within the scope of available resources, and to serve as the central point through which community needs are identified and actively addressed.
2. To operate the hospital on a financial basis that is self-sustaining from service charges yet equitable for patients and, when possible, reserving tax funds or alternative sources of revenues for capital expenditures or for the financing of care for clearly identified groups of patients.
3. To enable the hospital to meet requirements for licensing and certification, as appropriate, and to meet the standards of the Joint Commission on Accreditation of Hospitals.
4. To foster beneficial relationships among administration, governing board, medical staff, and employees, opposing unionization but encouraging enlightened and equitable personnel policies.
5. To keep the community informed of hospital needs and progress through the media and contact with local groups, and to cooperate fully with community organizations and agencies also involved with health and social needs.

Assisted by a start up grant from the Duke Endowment, CHHS first entered into management contract arrangements in October 1974. A potential market of 140 hospitals with fewer than 200 hospital beds in the two Carolinas was identified. The initial plan was to enter into contracts with two small hospitals in 1974 with an eye towards adding four other subscribers over a three year period. By the end of the first seven months, however, growth had accelerated to five hospitals under contract. This growth was accomplished without major marketing activity and at the requests of the contracting hospitals. These five hospitals comprised 235 beds and served an average of 170 patients per day.[12]

Buoyed by this initial success in attracting hospitals and aware that resources would be severely taxed by the unexpected growth, CHHS embarked on a program to expand and refine its Management Services division in 1975. The expansion went forth assisted by grant funding from the Duke Endowment and the W. K. Kellogg Foundation, the latter contributing $380,000 over a three year period for capital expenditures, other one time start up costs, unsubscribed capacity of core staff, and to maintain the flat rate charging structure for the five hospitals under contract until adjustments could be made. Grant assistance amounted to 37 percent of budgeted expenses of $950,000 for the first two years of operation. The remaining expenses were to be financed through contract fees. Financial self-sufficiency was expected by the conclusion of the third year, premised upon certain target figures for the number of hospitals and beds under contract.[13] Total service expansion was set at a target of sixteen hospitals.[14]

Implementation and Process

Aware of the sensitivities inherent in approaching an institution for the purposes of taking over its management functions, CHHS/MS used a restrained marketing strategy. No attempts were made to approach a hospital with the suggestion that existing management be forced out and CHHS/MS hired. Indeed, the decision to enter into a contract with a hospital was based primarily on CHHS's estimation of the commitment of the local board, community, and medical staff to address seriously their own problems.[15] Such an approach was used to minimize the potential for suspicion and conflict that accompanies fundamental change in an organization's operation. The early successes in attracting hospitals to the system reduced the necessity for aggressive marketing.

After establishing contact with a hospital, CHHS/MS develops a subscriber profile. The profile is developed by a CHHS/MS corporate support team with the assistance of a variety of personnel from the functional shared service divisions. The profile assesses the overall status of the hospital's operations and environment, and major problems and prospects for corrective action are identified. Not only is this step essential to protect CHHS/MS from entering an unmanageable situation, but it is also hoped that it will involve less orientation time for the new in-hospital director in the event a contract is signed. The shorter orientation span allows the hospital director to more rapidly reach full effectiveness, and should lead to early visibility of the benefits of the arrangement.[16] The criteria for accepting a hospital into an agreement are neither formalized nor hard and fixed. Factors such as public needs, expectations, and access are considered, in recognition of the corporation's public service mission, in addition to basic economic criteria.[17]

Once a new subscriber is signed, the CHHS/MS approach toward its management role has generally been to initiate the "fire fighting" measures needed to address the immediate serious problems found in many small rural hospitals. Installation of financial management systems and procedures follows. Efforts to improve community relations and apply core staff resources on the basis of priorities occurs during this early period.[18]

CHHS/MS's experience indicated that early education of trustees and medical staff leaders to the goals of the corporate management relationship was essential for making the initial major changes often required to reverse financial crisis and upgrade patient services.[19] Hence, care was taken to develop appropriate mechanisms toward this end. Continuing education seminars for local board members and, frequently, the medical staffs, were held at which topics such as the trustee's role in the modern hospital, local health issues, and national health care trends were addressed. A system Management Advisory Committee of the CHHS board provides a mechanism for guidance of system activities and for communication with client hospital boards.[20] A newsletter is published and sent to the trustees informing them of CHHS/MS activities. Trustees are also kept informed on a regular basis with periodic financial and other operating reports. Chief responsibility for trustee-medical staff liaison and trustee role development is held by development coordination specialists on the central CHHS staff.

CHHS/MS also found it important to institute mechanisms to market the management contract relationship to other important constituencies of the hospital: the community at large and employees. Public relations assistance from CHHS/MS core communications staff provides for local newspaper articles, hospital newsletters, and annual reports which, in many cases, were being prepared for the first time in the hospitals.

Marketing the management arrangement to employees serves to reduce the apprehension, fear, and potential conflict accompanying a change in management and also aids in increasing employee satisfaction. The basic mechanisms in achieving these ends include: personnel practices such as employee handbooks, orientation programs, clearcut hospital employee policies and lines of authority, job descriptions, and equitable wage and salary plans. CHHS/MS central staff work informally with department heads to train them in the use of new procedures and techniques, particularly in the areas of financial management and employee supervision. Employees are also encouraged to participate in training activities sponsored by both outside agencies and the other service divisions within CHHS.

Considerable attention is given to relationships with the many external agencies that have an impact upon hospitals. One example of the CHHS/MS approach toward relating to such groups has been their successful effort to persuade three local citizens and two inhospital directors to serve on the boards of the Health Systems Agencies. The President of CHHS was the 1978 chairman of the Governing Council of the AHA assembly of Shared Services and Programs, while a CHHS trustee serves as the Consulting Director of the AHA Center for Multihospital Systems. The origins of CHHS in the state hospital associations of North and South Carolina point toward an aptitude to deal effectively with a variety of agencies. The observations of a senior CHHS development coordinator are illustrative of this:

> Evidence that there is a practical working relationship [with these outside groups] is apparent in that most of the Management Services staff, the Executive Director of the corporation, and the staff in other CHHS divisions are on a first-name basis with those individuals in positions of power and authority in these various agencies. Because long association and friendships exist, problems which arise concerning our individual hospitals are effectively handled through personal contact and periodic visits. Moreover, as new hospitals are added and the corporate size continues to increase, the influence of CHHS will be strengthened with these agencies to the betterment of individual institutions. In addition, members of both state hospital associations and one state Blue Cross plan serve on the corporate board of trustees of CHHS. Through a mutual respect and confidence in both corporate and agency abilities, working relationships are being continually improved.[21]

Perhaps more than any other aspect of management, CHHS/MS puts considerable emphasis on the development of improved financial management systems. Indeed, the ability of any institution to achieve its potential in terms of patient care is in large part a function of its ability to manage its resources effectively and maintain financial viability. Judging from the emphasis given in the contracting hospitals, it is probably one of the most visible symptoms of the "management gap." The central staff of CHHS/MS includes several financial management professionals to oversee development and operations in this area. Standardized systems and model format were developed by CHHS/MS to provide reliable cost and use data for budget making, reporting, and control. Business office procedures are addressed with the implementation of standardized accounting and reporting formats, the same being true for credit and collection procedures. Assistance in interpreting third party payor regulation and reporting requirements is provided by the central staff. Systems analysis and management engineering services are provided by the central staff as well, with considerable assistance from the CHIP division.

One consequence of the CHHS/MS model which evolved without a large hospital/medical center or some other provider base was that CHHS had no computer base or existing data processing program upon which to build. Original strategy called for adapting a commercial data processing system to the CHHS/MS program. Initial efforts revealed, however, that no vendor system could cost-effectively meet the specific needs of the institutions managed by CHHS/MS. These hospitals were remote from professional and technical EDP support and did not possess the sophistication nor resources to support the considerable in-service education requirements necessary for substantial inhouse programming. The system developed by CHHS/MS, with additional grant funding from the Duke Endowment, combined inhospital minicomputer terminals and a remote shared service bureau in a distributive processing system that handles the fiscal management functions of accounts receivable, inpatient accounting, payroll, general ledger, accounts payable, and inventory control. The system is specific to the needs of smaller hospitals, providing only necessary reports.[22] From a marketing standpoint, the data processing service was seen as essential if larger hospitals (100 beds or more) needed to ensure the future stability of the system, were to be attracted to CHHS/MS.[23]

CHHS management and inhospital staff also encourage and guide hospital boards in the areas of long-range planning. Three contracting hospitals now are instituting formal long-range planning strategies and several others have instituted long-range planning committees at the board level.[24] Planning efforts are not necessarily geared to maintaining the status quo. A long-range planning evaluation for Tyrrell County Hospital in Columbia, North Carolina, a 29 bed hospital with a deteriorating facility and a shrinking medical staff, was completed with the cooperation of the Tyrrell governing board, the county government, and external planners. The evaluation focused on opportunities available to the community for high quality ambulatory care with links to nearby acute care facilities, rather than merely attempting to maintain the existing facility. The facility has since been closed and an ambulatory care project initiated through the Rural Health Initiative program instituted in its stead.[25]

The existing CHHS/MS organizational setup is the result of CHHS's examination of its internal structures and mechanisms as well as adaptation from other multi-institutional systems. Systemwide support services and line management of hospitals is the responsibility of the Vice President for Management Services. Between the Vice President and the inhospital directors are two Area Directors whose responsibilities are divided on a geographic basis. A Finance Director at the level of the Area Directors is soon to be added, supplementing financial management support currently being performed by two Area Financial Directors.[26] The roles of the inhospital directors and chief financial officers have been described. Support staff and functional services, increasingly organized on a regional basis, provide the following kinds of services:

1. Routine and recurring services carried out in hospitals on a continuing basis.
2. Special, defined projects for a particular hospital.
3. Assistance in identifying problems at a hospital, advising on the practicality and feasibility of various options for addressing them, and recommending solutions.
4. Development of component systems or programs in their particular area of expertise for use by all hospitals.[27]

Impact and Outcome

One indicator of CHHS/MS performance in the marketplace is their ability to attract hospitals into contract agreements. As of April 1979, 13 hospitals, comprising 920 acute beds and 170 skilled nursing beds, were under contract. Four management contracts have been terminated:[28] in one instance a hospital was closed, in another the hospital withdrew with CHHS's concurrence, retaining the inhospital director and certain shared services.[29]

Hospital governing board satisfaction is an indicator of acceptance of the CHHS system. Available reports demonstrate that trustees have reacted favorably to the program. Typical are the trustees of Lee County Hospital who made it clear that had they not signed the management contract with CHHS they probably would not have survived.[30] One progress report related the following:

> . . . local boards continue to give CHHS very positive recommendations when they are contacted by the boards of prospective subscribers to the program. In fact, these recommendations are probably the best marketing device; the board of one hospital directly influenced the board of another to investigate, consider, and engage our management services.[31]

Of 24 questionnaires returned by trustees in a survey by CHHS, 10 reported "substantial effect to date" in meeting most objectives, 10 more reported "some effect," and 2 noted "expect effect from efforts underway," and 2 could not be categorized.[32]

A potential source of conflict derives from the dual reporting responsibilities of the inhospital director both to the hospital governing board and CHHS/MS. However, several hospital boards have indicated no such problems had been experienced.[33] A CHHS/MS Area Director offered the following explanation:

> One factor contributing to the credibility [imputed to CHHS/MS] may be the board's assurance that the management staff intends to carry out its responsibilities outside the influence of local politics and special interests within the hospital.[34]

As anticipated, the management contract program was successful in attracting management expertise. Several reports, such as the following, are indicative of this:

> The inhospital directors employed by CHHS for the institutions under contract have been among the most capable of those currently available. There is increasing competition for inhospital directorships . . . [and] it is apparent that young M.H.A.'s are more than willing to consider multihospital management as a career option and avenue for advancement.[35]

There have, however, been expressions of concern by CHHS that ". . . in the absence of mid-sized hospitals to serve as 'stepping stones,' career ladders from inhospital administration to system management have been insufficient."[36]

The central role performed by physicians in health care institutions suggests that their support is crucial to the success of any management arrangement. There is evidence that such support exists in the CHHS managed institutions. A physician at Lee County Memorial Hospital in Bishopville, South Carolina had high praise for the improvement in quality of patient care accompanying the management contract. He related that prior to the contract patients were bypassing the hospital to seek care. According to him, the situation has been ". . . completely reversed . . . the difference between day and night."[37] One physician who joined a CHHS managed hospital stated that he was directly influenced by the stability of its management and his faith in the ability of CHHS to operate the hospital in a way that would make it useful to him and his patients.[38]

In addition to these direct expressions of satisfaction and support are some indirect signs, notably the assistance and participation of physicians in physician recruitment efforts. Such efforts may suggest that the physicians are becoming more involved in the system and more willing to fill a cooperative role.[39] Recruitment efforts have resulted in the addition of 16 primary care physicians for the system as a whole more than offsetting a loss of five such physicians.[40] Despite this, the need for physicians in system hospitals remains a major concern.

The recruitment of a Director of Nursing Services and institution of full RN nursing coverage for the first time in one institution is also noteworthy.[41] Also important are the addition of a respiratory therapy department, initiation of full-time emergency room coverage and interim physician coverage in one or more hospitals during the management contract period.[42] The achievement of a two year accreditation by one hospital following a period of conditional accreditation and a decrease in the number of deficiencies noted by state inspection agencies are further indications of quality related improvements.[43] Such accomplishments have led the President of CHHS to cite quality of care and service related improvements as the area of greatest achievement.[44]

Community support for the system was evidenced by increases in the number of volunteers and gifts.[45] The physician recruitment effort was spearheaded by community groups established especially for this purpose and to identify sources of funds for the effort. In one case, the city council of Bishopville appropriated funds for recruitment.[46]

In the area of financial management, results have been found favorable. Ratio analysis (current ratio, days cash available, days revenue in accounts receivable, working capital turnover, debt/capital, net profit margin, and net operating gain) performed on six hospitals under CHHS management for approximately two years revealed improvement in five of the six.[47] Two hospitals, under CHHS management for less than 18 months, showed net gains of $294,000, compared to a $70,000 loss, and $366,000, compared to a gain of $33,000, the previous year.[48] Another hospital reduced its loss from $256,000 to $215,000 in one year, despite the infusion of $325,000 in county contributions the previous year, a practice now discontinued.[49] Overall, profit/loss performance in nine hospitals has improved from a loss per patient day of $3.89 for the year prior to the management contract to a gain of $6.47 for the first full year of CHHS management.[50] Patient charges have increased in CHHS hospitals, the result of budgeting and rate setting practices intended to make patient services self-sustaining from patient revenues. Rates remain competitive, however, with other area hospitals. Budgets in all but the two most recently contracting hospitals for fiscal year 1979 show, in the aggregate, compliance with the Voluntary Effort for Cost Containment target for cost increases of 11.6 percent.[51]

The system's progress toward financial self-sufficiency has been dependent upon the course of marketing and service development. Original financial projections called for breakeven to be reached at a level of approximately 16 hospitals, with 1,200 beds, or an average of 75 beds per institution, and the level of service components included in the early contract package. It was recognized that the CHHS marketing approach (which concentrated on hospitals with administrative vacancies) would influence the timing and number of new contracts, and, in actual experience, the addition of new hospitals was slower than anticipated. At the same time, experience demonstrated the need for additional service features to serve existing subscribers and attract additional hospitals of larger size. Instead of radically altering existing contract fees to support the cost of additional service development and marketing, CHHS sought out additional substantial grant assistance and has used it for these enhancements. As further strategy CHHS began making gradual adjustments in fee schedules for existing contracts as the hospitals became more financially stable and marketing efforts have brought larger hospitals with higher volume into the contract fold. CHHS staff forecasts that the system will be financially self-sustaining (with existing services and methods of service delivery) in fiscal year 1978-79, provided that current year marketing targets are reached.[52]

On balance, then, it would appear that CHHS has achieved a number of economic, organizational, and manpower benefits within the context of the full management-without-ownership model.

REFERENCES

1. Latimer, Ben and Poston, Pat. "Multi-State, Multi-Service Corporate Model." *Topics in Health Care Financing*, 2:25-34, Summer 1976.
2. Ibid.
3. Ibid.
4. Latimer, Ben. "Developing Multi-hospital Arrangements: Some Practical Considerations," *Hospital Progress*, 57:62-67, October 1976.
5. Carolinas Hospital and Health Services, Inc., "CHHS Management Services System Self-Evaluation," January 1979.
6. Ibid.
7. Klicka, Karl S., M.D. "Field Notes: Carolinas Hospital and Health Services, Inc." Charlotte, NC, March 30-April 1, 1977."
8. Latimer, Ben. "Systems That Secure Resources Help Ensure Hospitals' Survival," *Hospitals: J.A.H.A.*, 51:57-58, 60-61, March 1, 1977.
9. Carolinas Hospital and Health Services, Inc., "CHHS Management Services . . ."
10. Latimer, "Systems That Secure Resources . . ."
11. Carolinas Hospital and Health Services, Inc., "CHHS Management Services . . . "
12. Carolinas Hospital and Health Services, Inc. "Proposal for Development and Expansion: CHHS Management Services Division." Submitted to W. K. Kellogg Foundation, August 1975.
13. Ibid.
14. DeVries, Robert A. *Program Notes:* W. K. Kellogg Foundation, October 1975.
15. Latimer, "Developing Multi-hospital Arrangements . . . "
16. Milburn, Jack. "The Small Hospital Under Multiple Unit Management, A Decade of Implementation: The Multiple Hospital Management Concept Revisited," *Report of the 1975 National Forum on Hospital and Health Affairs.*
17. Latimer and Poston, "Multi-State, Multi-Service Corporate Model."
18. Carolinas Hospital and Health Services, Inc., "Progress Report to W. K. Kellogg Foundation: CHHS Comprehensive Management Services, 11-1-75 to 10-31-76."
19. DeVries, *Program Notes* . . .
20. Carolinas Hospital and Health Services, Inc., "CHHS Management Services . . . "
21. Carolinas Hospital and Health Services, Inc., "Progress Report to W. K. Kellogg . . . 11-1-75 to 10-31-76."
22. Latimer, Ben. Letter to John M. Lowe, III, W. K. Kellogg Foundation, September 29, 1977.
23. Carolinas Hospital and Health Services, Inc., "CHHS Management Services . . . "
24. Ibid.
25. Carolinas Hospital and Health Services, Inc., "Progress Report: CHHS Comprehensive Management Services, 11-1-76 to 10-31-77."
26. Carolinas Hospital and Health Services, Inc., "CHHS Management Services . . . "

27. Poston, Pat. "Hospital Administration in the CHHS System" (unpublished).
28. Carolinas Hospital and Health Services, Inc., "CHHS Management Services . . . "
29. Carolinas Hospital and Health Services, Inc., "Progress Report to W. K. Kellogg . . . 11-1-75 to 10-31-76."
30. Klicka, "Field Notes: Carolinas Hospital . . . "
31. Carolinas Hospital and Health Services, Inc., "Progress Report to W. K. Kellogg . . . 11-1-75 to 10-31-76."
32. Carolinas Hospital and Health Services, Inc., "CHHS Management Services . . . "
33. Klicka, "Field Notes: Carolinas Hospital . . . "
34. Milburn, "The Small Hospital Under Multiple Unit Management . . . "
35. Carolinas Hospital and Health Services, Inc., "Progress Report to W. K. Kellogg . . . 11-1-75 to 10-31-76."
36. Carolinas Hospital and Health Services, Inc., "CHHS Management Services . . ."
37. Klicka, "Field Notes: Carolinas Hospital . . ."
38. Ibid.
39. Milburn, "The Small Hospital Under Multiple Unit Management . . ."
40. Carolinas Hospital and Health Services, Inc., "CHHS Management Services . . ."
41. DeVries, *Program Notes* . . .
42. Carolinas Hospital and Health Services, Inc., "Progress Report to W. K. Kellogg . . . 11-1-75 to 10-31-76."
43. Ibid.
44. Latimer and Poston, "Multi-State, Multi-Service Corporate Model."
45. Milburn, "The Small Hospital Under Multiple Unit Management . . ."
46. Klicka, "Field Notes: Carolinas Hospital . . ."
47. Carolinas Hospital and Health Services, Inc., "CHHS Management Services . . ."
48. Ibid.
49. Ibid.
50. Ibid.
51. Ibid.
52. Personal communication with Ben Latimer, President, CHHS, March 1, 1979.

Eastern Maine Medical Center— Brandow/Johnson Management Associates

Background and Structure

Eastern Maine Medical Center in Bangor, Maine has long been the clinical education and referral center in its service area. The 378 bed institution is the only large hospital in a service area that comprises more than one-quarter of the land area of New England and has a population of almost one-third million. The rural area is characterized by a dispersed but growing population, low per capita income, and hospitals of small size and limited finances. Situated in this environment and surrounded by many such hospitals, Eastern Maine was an early entrant into the development of shared clinical services, its regional pathology services originating about 30 years ago.

In recent years Eastern Maine expanded shared services in both clinical and administrative areas. Administrative services were offered in accounting, cost report preparation, and medical records, to name a few. A spirit of cooperation was nurtured between Eastern Maine Medical Center and area trustees, who were described as ". . . independent of mind and frugal . . . ."[1] The presidents of all surrounding hospital boards have accepted membership as incorporators of the Eastern Maine Medical Center—the group that elects the Eastern Maine governing board.[2] Trustees, physicians, and administrators from affiliated hospitals sit on the Eastern Maine Regional Services Advisory Council as well. Such mechanisms have built a base of support for continued close relationships between Eastern Maine and surrounding hospitals.

Management contracts were felt to be a logical extension of the shared services program and cooperative environment. The need was evident: almost two-thirds of the area hospitals were without the services of fully trained administrators.[3] Indeed, in each of the first four cases where Eastern Maine was approached concerning the possibility of a management contract, it was the administrator, recognizing a need for assistance, who initiated the contact.[4] Conversely, Eastern Maine had built up a considerable amount of administrative talent felt to be necessary to a large and self-sufficient hospital in a remote region: 10 administrative team members possessed management degrees at the master's level. Spurred initially by the interest of several hospitals in exploring a management contract relationship, Eastern Maine began the process of identifying the costs and benefits of such a program for all parties involved. The advantages identified for recipients, consistent with those commonly mentioned in the literature on the experience of multi-unit arrangements, included access to management expertise, economies of scale, and improved bargaining position with various external agencies. For the offering institution, a number of advantages were perceived:[5]

1. Eastern Maine would be better able to attract and retain persons of unusual expertise while at the same time spreading over a larger base the costs associated with such talent.
2. The opportunity existed to move in the area of multi-unit systems so as to build on existing relationships and referral patterns which focused on Eastern Maine Medical Center.
3. It provided the opportunity for managers and other personnel to benefit from a wide spectrum of experience with management tools and systems as well as a mechanism for continuing education, with the resultant improvement in performance and in patient care.
4. It would provide a broader base of strength with which to deal with legislative, regulatory, and planning bodies.

The Eastern Maine governing board had several concerns in deciding how best to respond to the perceived need for management contracts. One reservation was the possible overextension of existing management capability. Another issue related to keeping responsibilities clear and costs properly allocated and isolated. Of central concern from a marketing standpoint was how to avoid any fears of loss of autonomy on the part of the small community hospitals. Tax laws were yet another complicating matter. Regulations of the Internal Revenue Service specify that income resulting from trade or business conducted by a 501 (c) (3) organization that is not substantially related to the exercise of such an organization's charitable, educational, or other exempt purpose is taxable. Under one interpretation, the proceeds from management contracts could be considered as such unrelated-business income.[6] The only exception defined by the Tax Reform Act of 1976 would be for services performed for a tax-exempt facility, provided that services were consistent with that facility's tax-exempt status and that charges for services were based on reasonable cost. While possible that relief might be found in the 1976 Act, it was not clear how that law would be applied in this particular case.[7] In light of these considerations, the Eastern Maine board voted to form a wholly owned subsidiary corporation, reasoning that it would be the most flexible vehicle with which to pursue the management contract concept.

Such was the origin of Brandow/Johnson Management Associates, taking the names of Robert H. Brandow and John C. Johnson, the Executive Director and Administrator for Eastern Maine Medical Center, respectively. The subsidiary is a regular business corporation organized under the Maine Business Corporation Act and governed by a board comprised of trustees of Eastern Maine and the subsidiary's officers, Brandow and Johnson. Brandow/Johnson Management Associates report at least annually to the finance and executive commitees of the Eastern Maine board on the extent of its activities and its financial status. Its mission is limited to the provision of management services: all other shared services remain the province of the medical center. Several goals of the subsidiary were articulated:[8]

1. To assist nonprofit community hospitals to fulfill their respective hospital goals and service commitments.
2. To assist hospital boards of trustees to fulfill their eleemosynary and fiduciary responsibilities.
3. To enhance the quality of hospital management and thereby enhance the quality of hospital care.
4. To assist community hospitals to maximize their limited resources while minimizing their operational costs.

The management contracts entered into by Brandow/Johnson represent an application of the full-management-without-ownership model.

A Typical Contract

The contract agreement with the Down East Community Hospital, a 38 bed hospital in Machias, Maine, illustrates the typical contract.[9] Down East retains complete legal ownership and control of its facility, assets, and services. The managing organization may make no significant changes in hospital operations unless approved by the contracting hospital's governing board. Brandow/Johnson is charged with reporting periodically to the contracting board on the financial condition of the hospital, actions taken, recommended areas for improvement, and all other areas relevant to the health and progress of the hospital. Brandow/Johnson employees provide the services of a full-time administrator over whom the contracting board retains the right of approval before appointment. The administrator is responsible to the contracting board or its designated committees on all matters of local hospital policy, the implementation of such policy, and the execution of the budget as approved by the contracting board. The local board or Brandow/Johnson may remove the administrator at any time. In such an event, Brandow/ Johnson is obliged to render interim administrative coverage and recommend a replacement within 180 days upon penalty of contract termination. Brandow/Johnson is obligated to provide consultation services of its administrative officers and other Eastern Maine personnel as requested by the administrator. Consultations in areas such as credit and collections, dietary services, labor relations, purchasing, nursing, and materials management are envisioned. The contract is for a period of one year, renewing each year thereafter unless 90 day written notice of intention to terminate is provided by either party. Stipulation is made that no employee or former employee of Brandow/Johnson may be employed by a contracting hospital for a period of one year after a contract termination. It is apparent that numerous checks have been included to protect local autonomy.

The management fee has several components, which vary according to the needs of the institution. There is a basic fee which covers the recruitment and supervision of the administrator, the establishment of reporting and control mechanisms for the board, phone consultations, frequent attendance by Brandow/Johnson staff at board meetings, and all other shared services of the medical center. A separate fee for the salary of the administrator is charged as well as a percentage of that salary for fringe benefits and indirect expenses. All other consultation services when approved by the local board are provided and billed at an hourly rate based upon salary plus fringes and indirect expenses.[10]

The management contract program received initial grant support from the W. K. Kellogg Foundation amounting to $298,645 on a declining basis over three years beginning in mid-1977. The monies were to be applied to subsidize the management fee, related shared services, and some of the initial expense of the administrator. The grant subsidy was seen as important from a marketing standpoint in that the start-up costs rather than the long-run benefits of such contract agreements are more visible to potential clients. The grant was to be supplemented by expected revenues for the period. Targets of six contracts and financial self-sufficiency by the end of the grant period were established.[11]

Implementation and Process

Brandow/Johnson identified its primary service market to be those hospitals with at least 25 beds within reasonable driving time from Eastern Maine Medical Center. A total of 15 hospitals, comprising 1,145 short-term and 292 long-term beds, met this criteria. Another six hospitals with 378 short-term and 12 long-term beds were identified as a secondary market. Most of these institutions were already linked to Eastern Maine via shared clinical or administrative services.[12] Although certain stipulations of the grant restrict Brandow/Johnson from serving other than nonprofit institutions for the duration of the grant, it is envisioned that contracts with nursing homes may be sought in the future,[13] thereby adding an element of vertical integration to the system.

Contract development is considered a four phase process. The first phase involves a feasibility study once contact has been made and interest expressed by a potential client. The feasibility study includes a management audit, financial review, interviews with staff, and review of policies, procedures, and minutes of meetings, all designed to reveal whether a management contract would be of mutual benefit.[14]

The second phase begins with the presentation to the client's governing board of the feasibility study findings. If the board votes to accept the contract, Brandow/Johnson begins to screen applicants, and refer acceptable applicants for the administrator's position to the client board for their approval.[15]

The third phase involves the newly hired administrator and Brandow/Johnson staff in the development of a "Management Action Plan." This document builds upon and addresses those problems identified in the feasibility study and is presented to the client board for approval. The plan emphasizes program development, productivity, and long-range planning. It is designed to formalize the board's long-range planning and to strengthen communication between the board and management. The final phase encompasses the implementation of the plan, continuous evaluation, and periodic development and presentation of new management plans.[16]

Brandow/Johnson takes an active role in physician recruitment. A physician placement service and standardized physician contracts were developed in the grant's first year. Eastern Maine has a good track record in physician recruitment, having doubled its own active staff within a six year period. In 1977, for the first time, family practice residents completed training at Eastern Maine and it is hoped that this program, the only residency program sponsored by Eastern Maine, will be a source of new physicians in the area. The success of physician recruitment in these medically underserved areas is considered crucial to the success of the entire management contract program.[17]

Several activities serve to illustrate the kind of steps taken in contracting hospitals in the program's first year. A mock presurvey program has been designed and completed to prepare managed hospitals for licensure and accreditation surveys. A library of standard department policy and procedure manuals has been created. Efforts were undertaken to develop standardized productivity measures of hospitals and their departments. Periodic administrator's conferences have been held to promote the exchange of ideas and cost saving measures.[18]

An Executive Vice President with responsibilities solely in the management contract program was hired by Brandow/Johnson in the first year to handle a heavier than anticipated workload. In addition, a Vice President for Finance has been hired to manage systemwide fiscal affairs.

Impact and Outcome

Although the management contract program has been in existence for less than two years, there are several favorable indicators. Four hospitals signed contracts within the first 13 months: Down East Community Hospital, 38 beds; Mayo Memorial Hospital, 52 beds; Millinocket Community Hospital, 50 beds; and Castine Community Hospital, 14 beds. This result has exceeded the target timetable established in the grant. Even more encouraging has been the renewal of contracts by the Down East and Mayo Memorial hospitals, the first two contracting institutions.[19] Indeed, the early acceptance of the program and rapid growth have taxed existing resources to the extent that additional resources were recruited and a tactical adjustment made to de-emphasize marketing efforts in favor of attending to program development.[20]

Mayo Memorial Hospital has already seen a marked decrease in days of accounts receivable outstanding owing to the new management.[21] Observers also report a noticeable improvement in department head and employee morale.[22] Board members and medical staff at Down East have expressed "considerable enthusiasm" for the program, expecting it to match the favorable results of past shared clinical services.[23]

On balance, Eastern Maine appears to have been able thus far to demonstrate the potential of the wholly owned subsidiary approach to the management contract model. A number of checks have been put in place to protect local autonomy, which have served to enhance marketability of the program. It is believed that a solid base has been developed for future expansion of the system.

REFERENCES

1. Eastern Maine Medical Center. "Proposal by Eastern Maine Medical Center for a Hospital Contract Management Organization in Maine," draft, March 25, 1977.
2. Ibid.
3. Ibid.
4. Ibid.
5. Johnson, John C. Eastern Maine Medical Center. Letter and materials sent to Richard M. Meserve, Down East Community Hospital, March 21, 1977.
6. Letter from legal counsel to Robert H. Brandow, Eastern Maine Medical Center, January 10, 1977.
7. Ibid.
8. Brandow/Johnson Management Associates, Inc. "First Year Progress Report to the W. K. Kellogg Foundation," July 1978.
9. Draft of "Agreement for Hospital Management Services" between Brandow/Johnson Management Associates, Inc. and Down East Community Hospital.
10. Eastern Maine Medical Center, "Proposal by Eastern Maine Medical Center . . ."
11. Brandow, Robert A. Eastern Maine Medical Center. Letter and materials sent to Robert A. DeVries, W. K. Kellogg Foundation, April 14, 1977.
12. Eastern Maine Medical Center, "Proposal by Eastern Maine Medical Center . . ."
13. Letter from R. Brandow to Robert A. DeVries, May 18, 1978.
14. Johnson, Eastern Maine Medical Center. Letter and materials . . .
15. Ibid.
16. Ibid.
17. Eastern Maine Medical Center, "Proposal by Eastern Maine Medical Center . . ."
18. Brandow/Johnson Management Associates, Inc., "First Year Progress Report . . ."
19. Ibid.
20. Ibid.
21. Klicka, Karl S., M.D. Field Notes on visit to Eastern Maine Medical Center, November 28-30, 1977.
22. Ibid.
23. Ibid.

Fairview Community Hospitals, Inc.

Background and Structure

Fairview's first step into multi-unit health care institution arrangements began with the opening in 1965 of Fairview-Southdale Hospital. Located in Edina, Minnesota, Fairview-Southdale opened as a satellite of Fairview Hospital of Minneapolis. Following the consolidation with Lutheran Deaconess Hospital in 1973, the corporation took the name of Fairview Community Hospitals.[1]

Fairview began its experiment with multi-unit arrangements for many of the same reasons that are common to the origins of similar undertakings: to react to the call for quality medical care at a reasonable cost in an increasingly demanding regulatory and financial environment via an organizational system response. What was unique about Fairview's response, however, was the form it took. Looking to an organizational model found in the banking industry, Fairview adopted the holding company concept, envisioning it as a means of combining high quality top management, a wider capital base, and expanded central services, while retaining the advantages of local unit autonomy.[2] The holding company concept, as adapted to the health care setting by Fairview, is characterized by the pooling of assets and liabilities of previously independent institutions which then fall under the ownership and policy control of a single corporate governing board. In the Fairview system, the corporate board deals with broad policy questions related to long-range planning, financial supervision, and program coordination. A second characteristic of the holding company approach is the use of local operating boards that are responsible for the day-to-day operations of their individual hospital. Each hospital maintains its own separate medical staff and has its own administrator. In the Fairview model, the administrator, appointed by the local operating board on the recommendation of the Fairview president, reports directly to the president. Each hospital retains significant latitude on such important community concerns as the ethical-medical policies adopted to guide medical practice in its hospital.[3] The holding company approach was adopted in 1971 with the addition of Lutheran Deaconess' 278 beds to Fairview's 415 beds and Fairview-Southdale's 402 beds.

During this period, Fairview developed a plan whereby their corporate resources would be made available to hospitals in rural Minnesota and upper Midwest areas in an effort to assist these hospitals in improving their management capabilities and also to broaden Fairview's base. The result was the sale of data processing, central purchasing, and warehousing services to area rural institutions, referred to as "affiliated hospitals," on a variation of a shared services model.[4]

Encouraged by the increasing nationwide acceptance of multi-unit arrangements, and motivated by an overall strategy of corporate growth, their past successes in such arrangements, and by a healthy financial and managerial resource position, Fairview, in 1973-74, began a program to accelerate growth by increasing both the number of hospitals served and the range and depth of management relations with these hospitals.[5] At this stage, Fairview was operating the three owned "holding company" hospitals, and was engaged in selected management services with six other institutions. Total beds served amounted to 1,980.

Looking for assistance to fund this development, Fairview turned to the W. K. Kellogg Foundation. Total cost of expansion, promotion and implementation was budgeted at approximately $400,000 over a three year period. Kellogg funding amounted to $191,450 of this total. Revenues from services were expected to fund an increasing proportion of the total budget through the period while grant funding was to be distributed on a declining basis. Full internal self-support was targeted by the fourth year.[6]

As part of this growth program, Fairview initiated the development and implementation of a full management contract program. Thus, opportunities for hospitals to join the Fairview system were available at three levels of participation:

1. The fully owned and managed "holding company" hospital level
2. The full management contract without ownership level
3. The selected management services level

The structure of the full ownership level has been described. Fairview perceived the advantages of this level to be the ability to better integrate planning efforts and achieve greater control over financial operations while maintaining a fairly high level of local autonomy.

The structure of the full management contract provides for Fairview to assume total management responsibility for the daily operations of the contracting hospital. Ownership and policy control remain in the hands of the local governing board, to which Fairview reports. The incumbent administrator may or may not be retained. Any new administrator is appointed jointly by the local governing board and Fairview. The administrator's salary is paid by Fairview. The contract fee is established on either a percentage of gross revenues or a flat fee basis, and its magnitude is a function of the quantity of services necessary to achieve the hospital's goals. The contracting institution, through its administration, may make use of Fairview corporate staff and central corporate services as needed.[7]

Fairview identified the full management contract level as either an intermediate step in a progression to full ownership, should that become mutually desirable, or as an end point in itself. From the viewpoint of Fairview, it provides an opportunity to evaluate the hospital in terms of desirability for future ownership and an opportunity to improve Fairview's management systems through on-site experience. For the community hospital, Fairview feels that it provides the same opportunity to evaluate the desirability of further ties without significant risk, as well as providing the community access to resources not usually available, thereby strengthening the hospital.[8]

The third level, shared services agreements, involves the least commitment. There are available to each affiliate a broad array of available services, as indicated below:

Administration	Finance and Accounting
Business Office	Housekeeping
Clinical Laboratory	Marketing
Data Processing	Materials Management
Dietary	Medical Education
Facilities Planning	Medical Library

Medical Records	Pharmacy Management
Nurse In-Service	Planning
Education	Public Relations
Nursing Service	Respiratory Therapy
Personnel	Management
	Utilization Review

Specialists from these various departments are available to consult with the affiliates on a one-time or continuing basis.[9] Fairview saw this level as an entry step to further working relationships, holding advantages for both participants similar to those outlined in the full management contract level.[10]

To further the goals of growth in the number of institutions served and expansion of services offered, several priorities and subgoals were established. First priority was to be given to the development and implementation of the full management contract level. A target of 8 to 12 hospitals under the total management and/or ownership options was established in this regard. The addition of 250 institutional beds each year under shared services arrangements was targeted for the third level of participation. The primary focus in terms of expansion of available services was to be in the areas of financial management, accounting, and business office management.[11]

A minimum three year commitment was set as a requirement under any option. Fairview felt that this depth of involvement was necessary to allow meaningful medium and long-range planning at the corporate level.[12]

In sum, the structure built by Fairview seems well designed to achieve its strategy of corporate growth and service mission. The unique combination of well-defined levels of participation, involving progressively higher stages of system commitment, is viewed as a significant step in overcoming the apprehension which often serves as a barrier to cooperative ventures designed to deal with the serious resource problems faced by small rural community hospitals.

Implementation and Process

Along with the decision to pursue an ambitious growth strategy and deepen the commitment of participating institutions via the full management contract option came the realization that an aggressive marketing strategy must be adopted.[13] Previously, Fairview had only served those who came to them with requests for help. Among the tools used at that time were such common ones as printed brochures and visual presentations.[14] One fresh approach was the development of a model that defined the type and cost of services that a typical hospital entering into a contract with Fairview would experience.[15] The potential market is seen to be hospitals in the upper Midwest with fewer than 175 beds, many of which have no working relationships with any of the several major hospital groups in Minnesota.[16]

Once an acceptable agreement is reached between Fairview and another institution, the plan calls for an implementation team whose task it is to evaluate the requirements for services and install the needed management systems. The team is composed of an administrator, a systems analyst, a financial manager, and a materials coordinator. The team is to have major educational responsibilities in relation to the hospital's board, medical staff, and department heads.[17]

Communication between Fairview and the participating institutions takes place through a variety of vehicles. Affiliate hospital administrators and controllers are brought together for review and discussion of shared services programs. Administrators in owned and managed institutions participate in weekly management meetings. Yearly trustee/administrator seminars are held which have included presentations from university program faculty on such topics as multihospital systems, capital financing, and health manpower. Education and training for department heads and department staff are accomplished in one of two ways: either Fairview staff go to individual hospital sites to assist in specific training programs at the sites or the community hospital personnel visit Fairview to participate in the variety of in-service programs offered there. These more formal vehicles are, of course, in addition to the informal channels of communication that develop, and supplementary to the management reporting systems that are established.

Fairview's main focus in its managed hospitals has been in the fiscal management area. Assistance has been given to improve budgeting, forecasting, rate setting, reimbursement, cost accounting, business office management, productivity control, inventory management, and capital purchase analysis—in sum, any and all areas relating to the fiscal health of the institution. A review of the specifics of some of the programs illustrates this involvement:[18]

- Productivity standards were developed for the nursing staff of a managed hospital, defining maximum staffing levels for each level of occupancy. Following each payroll period, nursing hours per patient day are computed and compared to the standards, and reported to administration together with explanation of variations.

- A new chart of accounts at managed hospitals was revised and implemented with an expanded number of subaccounts for increased control of departmental expenses.
- A financial accounting system, not requiring a computer system, was developed for use at small managed hospitals. The system produces a separate income statement for each department and compares monthly and year-to-date variances of actual to budgeted levels for each subaccount.
- A methodology was developed for capital equipment inventories and provided to hospitals along with assistance in the planning and supervision of the inventory process.
- Study and review of business office procedures was undertaken in the managed hospitals, leading to reassignment of work duties, establishment of internal control procedures, and recommendations on methods to improve accounts receivable by developing formal credit, claims processing, and credit follow-up policies.
- A comprehensive budgeting assistance and education process was introduced in the managed hospitals, ranging from the projection of departmental activity levels, cost finding, and rate setting, to the preparation and presentation before the Minnesota rate review panel. The process calls for significant involvement by Fairview staff in the first year of management and the assumption of responsibility for the process by the hospital staff in subsequent years.
- The Fairview central personnel department develops standardized wage and salary programs, personnel policies, and benefit programs for use in the managed institutions.

While the main focus has been that of fiscal management, assistance is available to managed and affiliated hospitals alike in any of the service areas outlined earlier.

Fairview was able to implement the total management contract in two institutions during the three year grant period. The first hospital, Princeton Community Hospital, provides an illustration of the type institution for which the total management contract arrangement is an attractive option. Located 50 miles north of Minneapolis, this 39 bed acute care hospital found itself, in the words of one observer, with:

> ... one ... chairman of the board, one chief of medical staff, five doctors, expenditures that surpassed income, and an administrator's office door that had to swing both ways to accommodate the constant flow of occupants.[19]

On top of this, there was considerable community dissatisfaction with the hospital's plight and the chairman of the board and chief of staff were not on speaking terms.[20] On the initiative of the medical staff, the hospital approached Fairview and signed a three year management contract in 1975.[21] The incumbent administrator resigned at this point and a new individual, experienced in small hospital management, assumed the administrator's position.[22]

The second hospital, the Waseca Area Memorial Hospital, entered into a management contract in 1976 on the vote of the administrator, medical staff, and Waseca City Council (the governing board). Waseca Memorial, a 35 bed hospital 75 miles north of Minneapolis, had problems similar to those of Princeton, except that the financial situation was more serious: losses had been experienced in six of the last seven years, including a $119,000 loss from operations in the year prior to the management contract. In this instance, the incumbent administrator was retained.[23]

Thus, the process by which Fairview addresses the management problems in member hospitals is characterized by a variety of channels for communication and exchange between participants and a heavy focus on financial analysis and control.

Impact and Outcome

An explicit objective of the grant funding provided by the W. K. Kellogg Foundation was to evaluate the performance of the major management services provided by Fairview.[24] Fairview staff devoted considerable attention to this end, utilizing methodologies reviewed by outside experts. Specific evidence of outcomes are therefore more readily available than in many other systems. In addition, Fairview has received substantial notice and scrutiny from a number of groups who have contributed to the measurement of Fairview's endeavors. The Harvard University Graduate School of Business has selected Fairview as the focus of a case study for teaching purposes, describing Fairview as "an effective organization of hospitals."[25]

The Health Services Research Center of the Hospital Research and Educational Trust, in conjunction with Northwestern University, provided an overview of the management performance of Fairview which indicated the following:

> ... The relative reduction in cost and price for system F (Fairview) apparently resulted from realized economies of scale in all operational areas. The system's administrative costs per case fell 20.2

percent over the period relative to that of its control set and its hotel services cost fell 7.5 percent . . . The savings were the result, in large part, of the system's lower growth rates in several areas of administrative expense and in man-hours worked in hotel services . . .

Finally, the data indicated that, although the margin between the price and cost of services provided was the same for the system and its control set at the beginning of the period, the system's margin declined over the period relative to that of its control set. This finding provides evidence that the system benefited the community it served not only through the provision of relatively equal health services at lower relative prices but also by operating with a relatively smaller margin of revenues over expenses.[26]

A study performed by the accounting firm of Coopers and Lybrand rated the Fairview data processing system highly in both quality of output and unit cost.[27] A comparison with a study done by Advanced Health Systems, which measured costs of financial data processing, revealed that costs were significantly lower in the Fairview system despite the fact that Fairview's costs included many nonfinancial elements, such as laboratory and medical records. Estimated annual savings for the three owned hospitals from this cost difference amounted to $200,000.[28]

Fairview staff studies revealed that hospitals utilizing the Fairview system have reduced their accounts receivable days outstanding by a minimum of ten days during a three year period.[29] Another staff study revealed positive results from the materials management program. Sampling studies showed savings of from 10 to 30 percent from group purchasing. Comparison with another large group purchasing organization of items representing 28 percent of Fairview's inventory showed gross savings of 14 percent.[30]

One notable example of financial benefit accruing to a hospital participating at the shared service level resulted from a review of previous year's Medicare cost reports of the hospital by Fairview financial staff. Reimbursement of from $10,000 to $14,000 that would otherwise have been lost was realized by the review, and changes implemented in the cost report preparation have resulted in approximately $6,000 in savings in each subsequent year.[31]

Overall results at Princeton Community Hospital, the first of the full management contract hospitals, were equally impressive, particularly in terms of financial and productivity indicators:[32]

- Nurse staffing procedures that were implemented lowered nurse FTEs per patient day by approximately 12 percent during the grant period and the mix of RNs, LPNs, and nurse aides was shifted to less costly levels with no evidence of quality reductions. Estimates indicated that if precontract staffing levels had been maintained, nurse salary costs would have been $15,000 per year higher.

- A decrease in accounts receivable turnover of 19 days was realized, translating into a $30,000 increased cash flow.
- Inventory per bed levels were decreased by 12 percent for an estimated savings of $5,000.
- Total savings in audit fees amounted to $3,000 per year.
- An arrangement reached for the sharing of a physical therapist with a local nursing home saved $6,000 initially and $900 annually thereafter.
- A net gain from operations was achieved for the first time in four years during the first year of the full management contract whereas the budget had called for a $38,000 loss. A $58,000 net gain was achieved the following year.

General quality of care indicators showed positive results as well:
- JCAH accreditation was applied for and received on a full two year basis; in the previous twenty-one years, Princeton Hospital had never been accredited.
- Medical service clinics were opened in urology, general surgery, and orthopedics.
- Nursing audits were begun for the first time.
- A member of the medical staff reported improvements in patient care and increased nursing staff morale.
- A community shortage of two physicians was relieved within one year.

These illustrations of improvement were underscored with the decision of the Princeton governing board to request membership in the Fairview system on an ownership basis prior to the end of the second year of the management contract. The request was accepted by the Fairview board and ratified by the community membership of Princeton Hospital.[34]

The second management contract hospital, Waseca Area Memorial Hospital, although only under management contract beginning with the final year of the grant period under study, exhibited significant early progress:[35]
- For the first time in seven years, Waseca realized an operating gain.
- In the first eleven months of operation its accounts receivable turnover dropped from 90 to 65 days, representing an increased cash flow of $61,000.

- Whereas in the nine months prior to the contract Waseca had borrowed a total of $125,000 from the City of Waseca to maintain operations, no money had been borrowed since the contract went into effect.

In the words of one observer, discussing the situation at Waseca with members of the board, medical staff, and the administrator, there was ". . . a complete turnaround from a very unsatisfactory situation that had existed prior to the . . . management contract."[36]

At the end of the grant period, Fairview owned four hospitals, managed one under the management contract option, and provided specific management services to eleven affiliated institutions, one of which was a nursing home. Total beds served amounted to 3,003.[37] This may be compared to the situation at the outset, in which there were three owned hospitals, no management contracts, and six shared service institutions, totaling 1,980 beds. Shortly after the grant period another management contract was signed with a municipal hospital in Ortonville, Minnesota.[38] Compared to the ambitious plans for growth, Fairview fell somewhat short of its goals. In particular, they had not been as successful as was hoped in adding management contracts. The factor of community and institutional pride was identified as the main barrier in instances where discussions took place but in which no contract arrangement was reached.[39] To address this problem, Fairview planned stepped-up marketing efforts.[40] It may be that as Fairview's experience with hospitals under management contracts becomes more well known, and to the extent that the results are positive, hospitals may be more willing to enter into contracts. Indeed, Waseca's decision to contract with Fairview was clearly influenced by the benefits it saw at Princeton.[41]

Plans established at the end of the grant period called for a continuation in the growth of each level of participation and the implementation of a new strategy described as the "Key Hospitals" concept. As envisioned, the "Key Hospitals" would be major facilities in their geographic regions, operating at about 100 beds, possessing a healthy financial and management situation, and lying in a "natural catchment area." With assistance from Fairview, these institutions would become regional supply and specialty centers in the areas of clinical services, finance and management skills, and shared services. The "Key Hospitals" would in turn serve small local community hospitals where it is uneconomical for Fairview to serve directly. The resulting network would attempt to capitalize on common geographic characteristics, existing referral patterns and HSA planning areas, along with common social, ethnic, political, and economic backgrounds.[42] This concept, a variation of which is also being developed at Health Central, represents a promising extension of multi-institutional systems organized along regional lines.

REFERENCES

1. Hofstad, Paul A. Fairview Community Hospitals, "Annual Report Presented to W. K. Kellogg Foundation, September 1977."
2. Platou, Carl and Rice, James. "Multihospital Holding Companies," *Harvard Business Review,* 50:14-16, 18, 20-21, 146, 148-49, May-June 1972.
3. Ryan, Ann K. "The Fairview Phenomenon." *Corporate Report,* June 1976.
4. Hofstad, Fairview Community Hospitals, "Annual Report, 1977."
5. "The Fairview Community Hospitals Strategy for External Corporate Growth." April 1974.
6. DeVries, Robert A. *Program Notes:* "Fairview Community Hospitals, Inc." W. K. Kellogg Foundation, 1974.
7. Hofstad, Paul A. Letter to Karl S. Klicka, M.D., December 27, 1977.
8. "The Fairview Community Hospitals Strategy . . .
9. Hofstad, Fairview Community Hospitals, "Annual Report, 1977."
10. "The Fairview Community Hospitals Strategy . . .
11. DeVries, *Program Notes:* Fairview Community Hospitals, Inc."
12. Ibid.
13. "The Fairview Community Hospitals Strategy . . .
14. DeVries, *Program Notes*: "Fairview Community Hospitals, Inc."
15. Hofstad, Paul A. Fairview Community Hospitals, "Site Visit Progress Report Presented to K. S. Klicka, M.D., May 1977."
16. "Supplemental Information for the Fairview Community Hospitals Grant Request." 1974.
17. DeVries, *Program Notes*: "Fairview Community Hospitals, Inc."
18. Hofstad, Fairview Community Hospitals, "Site Visit Progress Report . . .
19. Ryan, "The Fairview Phenomenon."
20. Ibid.
21. Klicka, Karl S., M.D. "Field Notes: Fairview Community Hospitals, Minneapolis, Minnesota, May 8-10, 1977."
22. Edmands, Clay D. Fairview Community Hospitals, "Annual Report Presented to W. K. Kellogg Foundation, September 1975."
23. Edmands, Clay D. Fairview Community Hospitals, "Annual Report Presented to W. K. Kellogg Foundation, September 1976."
24. Ibid.
25. Ryan, "The Fairview Phenomenon."
26. "Multihospital Systems: An Evaluation," Chicago: Health Services Research Center of the Hospital Research and Educational Trust and Northwestern University, 1975.
27. Edmands, Fairview Community Hospitals, "Annual Report 1975."
28. Ibid.
29. Edmands, Fairview Community Hospitals, "Annual Report 1976."
30. Edmands, Fairview Community Hospitals, "Annual Report 1975."
31. Hofstad, Fairview Community Hospitals, "Annual Report 1977."
32. Hofstad, Fairview Community Hospitals, "Site Visit Progress Report . . ."

33. Annual Reports to the W. K. Kellogg Foundation, 1975-76-77.
34. Edmands, Fairview Community Hospitals, "Annual Report 1976."
35. Hofstad, Letter to Karl S. Klicka, M.D.
36. Klicka, "Field Notes: Fairview Community Hospitals."
37. Hofstad, Fairview Community Hospitals, "Annual Report 1977."
38. Hofstad, Letter to Karl S. Klicka, M.D.
39. Edmands, Fairview Community Hospitals, "Annual Report 1975."
40. Klicka, Karl S., M.D. Memorandum to Robert A. DeVries, May 16, 1977.
41. Edmands, Fairview Community Hospitals, "Annual Report 1976."
42. "Operating Center Plan: Managed and Affiliated Division," Fairview Community Hospitals, August 10, 1977.

Henry Ford Hospital

Background and Structure

The Henry Ford Hospital has long been recognized as a prestigious and innovative institution. The closed group practice of full-time salaried staff physicians at Henry Ford, a significant departure from the norm when it was instituted and still a relatively unusual one. It is one of the most visible examples of its inclination to experiment with and adopt progressive ideas in the delivery of medical care to the Greater Detroit area. In addition to its wide ranging patient care activities, Henry Ford Hospital also devotes substantial resources to medical research and health professional education. The resources and operating statistics of the institution are impressive: in 1974, when it began activities in multi-institutional arrangements, the hospital operated 1,015 beds in eight buildings on a 20 acre main campus in Detroit; employed 4,500 non-medical staff, 230 staff physicans, and 330 interns and residents; operated on a $120 million annual budget; recorded 26,867 admissions; possessed assets of $200 million; and was embarking on a $300 million renovation and building program.[1]

It was in this context that development of the Henry Ford Hospital Health Care System began. The potential for such a system was indicated by way of the numerous requests for assistance and advice from other health care institutions in Michigan to which Henry Ford had responded to the extent that its then existing organizational structure and resources permitted.[2] In studying the need and opportunity for the development of the system, Henry Ford reached the following conclusions that form both the basic rationale behind its decision to move forward with the system proposal and a statement of the particular strengths that the organization could offer:

> The nongovernmental, nonprofit hospitals form a logical base for the development of a 'system' of institutions and services. Characteristically they have:
> 1. Managerial talent
> 2. Financial resources
> 3. Medical leadership
> 4. Community roots
>
> The nongovernmental, nonprofit hospitals are especially well suited to demonstrate innovation and to seize the initiative in the development of a revised institutions network. They tend to avoid some of the major limitations experienced by public hospitals, academic health science centers, and the proprietaries.[3]

In establishing the system, six objectives were listed:[4]
1. To strengthen the voluntary, nongovernmental sector of health services delivery system.
2. To improve the coordination among various institutions.
3. To reduce unnecessary duplication and fragmentation of services.
4. To improve the accessibility of health services.
5. To increase the capability of delivering comprehensive health services.
6. To enhance the educational and research programs of Henry Ford Hospital.

From the perspective of the Henry Ford Hospital, in addition to enhancing its educational and research programs, the system would supplement and strengthen the network of clinical contacts and referrals.[5] The latter was of particular interest to Henry Ford given its extensive involvement in tertiary care with an exclusively hospital based medical staff.

Complementing these legitimate internal interests was a sense of responsibility, expressed by Executive Vice President Stanley Nelson, for an institution of Henry Ford's stature to serve the Greater Detroit and Michigan community by way of improving the management of small hospitals, thereby exerting a positive influence on the patient care services offered.[6]

The system proposed called for several different programs to achieve the objectives outlined above.

The core of the system was to be the continued operation of the existing main hospital and clinics, including emergency and unscheduled walk-in service.

The second element involved three satellite clinics serving suburban Detroit communities. The West Bloomfield Center, 20 miles from the main hospital, was built in 1975. Designed for initial service as an ambulatory facility, the Center was also viewed as the potential location of a satellite inpatient facility. The Troy Hemodialysis and Mental Health Clinics, built in 1973 and located 20 miles from the main hospital, serves as an outpatient treatment facility. The Fairlane Center in Dearborn was built in 1975 and serves as an ambulatory facility for a variety of primary care and specialty clinics.

The third element in the system called for programs to serve Detroit inner city populations. The Pallister-Lodge Clinic treats substance abuse patients, the Pelham Health Station offers primary care and referral services, the CHASS (Community Health and Social Services) Clinic serves a primarily Spanish-speaking community, and the Woodrow Wilson Clinic provides maternal and child health services. In addition, Henry Ford has combined with other Detroit health care institutions to provide shared preventive health education to inner city residents.

The fourth element called for further affiliation with other hospitals, nursing homes, and ambulatory care centers.

A fifth called for the extension of educational services.

The final element involved the extension of management services to other institutions via management contracts, shared services, and consultations.

Direction and development of the network, which came to be known as the Institutional Services Program, was provided by the creation of a separate division within Henry Ford called the Division of Institutional Services. An experienced health care administrator, reporting to Henry Ford executive officers, was hired to head the division. Development support for the division, with particular focus on the management services element, was sought and received from the W. K. Kellogg Foundation. The grant support amounted to $188,600 on a three year declining basis, or roughly 75 percent of an anticipated $255,000 budget for the division during the period. The remainder was to be financed by service fees, with a goal of complete financial self-support by the end of the three years.[7]

Initial market assessments and resource considerations were such that a decision was made to place limitations on the number and location of institutions to be served: the institutions were to be within 300 miles of Detroit; only three management contracts per year would be arranged, with a maximum of nine over the three year period; no more than six consultation contracts would be undertaken at any given time with growth limited to two per year.[8]

As to the content of services offered, Henry Ford envisioned that the services would be tailored to meet the needs of the contracting institution while efforts would be made to develop programs of service which would easily be adapted to a variety of institutions and situations. A typical contract would detail the services to be provided, responsibilities, relationships, duties, authority, length, termination conditions, and compensation.[9]

Under the full management contract option, three levels of management services were available. The "management services" level includes the provision of a full-time executive director and a full-time assistant director. Under "consultation services," the second level, assistance would be given by Henry Ford Hospital in such administrative areas as accounting, budgeting, and data processing, and in clinical services such as nursing and laboratory. The third level, "special studies," covers in-depth studies of selected problems or projects not covered under the above categories, e.g., a financial feasibility study of a proposed capital expansion project.

The responsibilities and relationships outlined provide that the full-time director and assistant director will be employees of and be paid by the Henry Ford Hospital. All other personnel remain employees of the contracting institution. The director and assistant director are appointed by Henry Ford's Executive Vice President with the consultation and advice of the governing board of the contracting institution. The appointed director is directly responsible to that governing board and performs all duties customarily performed by the chief executive officer of the institution. The local contracting institution retains all rights and obligations of ownership, with Henry Ford acting as an independent contractor, assuming no debts or liabilities of the institution.

The agreements were designed to be in force for three years, extending automatically at the end of the original term and each year thereafter for a period of one year, unless a 90 day termination notice is given by either party.

The management services fee, established for an annual period, requires the mutual consent of all parties and is billed and payable on a monthly basis. Consultation services are charged on a per diem basis with a budget for such services prepared annually by the hospital director for approval by the respective governing boards.

Implementation and Process

Aware of the apprehensions and sensitivities inherent in the development of interinstitutional ties between a large sophisticated urban institution and the small community hospital, Henry Ford Hospital decided on a relatively restrained approach in marketing its Institutional Services Program, in particular the full management contract option. This decision called for consultation agreements and full management contracts to be considered *only* on the invitation of hospital boards of trustees and/or chief executive officers.[10] Despite difficulty in attracting full management contracts, Henry Ford maintained this policy, reasoning that:

> In order to preserve our credibility and trust with administrators, we continue to be reluctant to approach hospital boards concerning contract management until we learn of an impending vacancy in the administrator's position.[11]

It would be misleading, however, to characterize the marketing strategy as a passive one. Considerable effort was exerted in promoting the visibility of the Institutional Services Program through a variety of avenues. News announcements conveying the purposes and resources available were sent to community newspapers throughout Michigan, to health care journals, to the Michigan Hospital Association, and to area hospital councils. Personal letters were sent to the chief executive officers of many hospitals in the state, informing them of opportunities for participation. The Administrator for Institutional Services recorded 105 visits in the first year of the program to small nonteaching hospitals, and participated in numerous hospital group conferences.[12]

Requests for assistance come to the Administrator for Institutional Services or to other Henry Ford staff through informal professional networks. At the invitation of the chief executive officer of the requesting institution, a visit to the facility is made by the Administrator for Institutional Services and a resource person familiar with the problem area. The problem is defined, the methodology and implementation schedule established, cost estimates made, and measurement tools devised.[13]

The experience of the Institutional Services Program followed a course somewhat different from what had been anticipated and planned, with no full management contracts signed in the three year period. During the first year, informal requests continued and increased in number, which was attributed to the growing awareness of Henry Ford's willingness to offer assistance as evidenced by the establishment of the Institutional Services Program. Henry Ford decided to continue to respond to these informal requests in the hope that more formal commitments would evolve from the relationships.[14] As this strategy progressed, three areas of activity came to comprise the content of the Institutional Services Program: (1) short-term assistance along the lines of the "consultation services" described above; (2) a broad range of assistance within a single institution, which approached but did not reach, the full management contract level; and (3) the initiation of a consortium of eight hospitals, including Henry Ford, located in southern Michigan.[15]

The short-term specific assistance activities involved both general administrative areas and clinical services. For example, the billing, data processing, and operations analysis departments of Henry Ford Hospital assisted the Community Health Center of Branch County in the formation of improved electronic data processing and accounting systems.[16] The administrator for Institutional Services and the Assistant Administrator for Business at Henry Ford reviewed the patient charge systems at Otsego Memorial Hospital in Gaylord, Michigan which led to the development of control procedures for charges initiating in the various departments of the hospital.[17] Hackley Hospital in Muskegon received the help of the program in selecting a new chief executive officer as did Wyandotte General Hospital in their attempt to identify factors that would lead to the employment and retention of a qualified nursing director.[18] Additional assistance included management engineering, nurse scheduling, personnel policy revision, fire and safety inspection consultations, and a considerable amount of in-service education and supervisory development programs.[19]

Various kinds of assistance were provided in the clinical service and quality of care areas on a short-term and/or continuing basis. A survey and resulting recommendations on operating room facilities, policies, and procedures were provided to Lansing General Hospital.[20] Through the Institutional Services Program, an agreement was reached whereby the medical staff and facilities of Henry Ford Hospital were utilized to provide routine and episodic care to the Southgate Residential Training Center, a Michigan Department of Mental Health Institution for the mentally retarded.[21] The Henry Ford Cardiovascular Disease Division Chairman and Electrocardiogram Department staff developed a computer assisted ECG interpretation and telephone consultation service that was utilized by many Detroit area health care providers.[22] At the request of local medical staffs in communities throughout the state, senior medical staff from Henry Ford provided numerous continuing medical education courses.[23] Other examples of assistance included in-service education for the respiratory therapy technicians and staff of North Detroit General Hospital, assistance in the development of effective medical audit procedures, EEG training, and the lending of a physician therapist and CCU Director.[24]

The second main area of program involvement related to the unique development of a broad range of continuing assistance to a single institution, the River District Hospital in St. Clair, Michigan. During the three year period, Henry Ford staff worked closely with River District in a variety of areas.[25] An eight week supervisory development program for first line managers at River District was led by Henry Ford's Administrator for Personnel. Henry Ford loaned a Director of Nursing to River District who reported to the River District Administrator while remaining on the Henry Ford payroll, and a similar agreement was reached to provide River District with a personnel director on a long-term basis. In time, River District employed their own Personnel Director who continued the consultative relationship with the Henry Ford Personnel Director. Respiratory therapy staff traveled to Henry Ford for in-service education programs, and consultation concerning the River District facility, program, and policies was provided. River District also participated in the computerized ECG and continuing medical education programs. In many ways this represented the closest approximation to a full management contract agreement experienced during the period.

The third major area of effort consisted of the initiation and formalization of a consortium of eight Southern Michigan hospitals that came to be known as Consolidated Hospital Resources. Other than Henry Ford and one other moderately sized institution, the participating hospitals were small hospitals (less than 100 beds) with limited resources. The stated purpose of the affiliation was to:

> . . .provide a vehicle through which participating hospitals voluntarily share resources or, through combined efforts, develop new ones in order to improve or expand capabilities and services offered to the hospitals' various communities.[26]

Direction of policy and program development and implementation rested with a steering committee comprised of the administrators of the eight participants. This committee engaged in a survey process with the staff assistance of a graduate student from the University of Michigan Program in Hospital Administration in order to identify likely program possibilities and develop feasibility studies of those projects. Early experimentation in jointly sponsored educational programs resulted in the formal development of an in-service and continuing education program that included a $30,000 annual budget supported by the participating hospitals. An educational coordinator was hired through Henry Ford who, under the guidance of the steering committee, became responsible for the design and implementation of the educational programs in the hospitals. Among the programs conducted were a reimbursement workshop for administrators and financial staff conducted by Henry Ford's assistant controller, and a critical care nursing course. An additional feature of Consolidated Hospital Resources was the establishment of consortiumwide advisory committees, in areas such as nursing, maintenance, and physical therapy, which met to share ideas and information and to further facilitate determination of educational program needs.[27]

Impact and Outcome

Perhaps the most disappointing aspect of the grant period was the inability to attract any full management contracts. Three prospective arrangements were scuttled for several different reasons. First, a hospital identified as a good candidate proved to be more interested in being acquired by Henry Ford than in developing a contractual relationship.[28] A second institution, in the final stages of coming to an agreement, withdrew from the negotiations as a result of opposition from its medical staff. The staff objected to having been left out of the negotiation process and feared that an eventual complete takeover might result, bringing with it the introduction of a full-time salaried medical staff similar to that at Henry Ford Hospital.[29] Henry Ford rejected a third hospital when it failed to be approved by a local comprehensive health planning agency.[30]

Several reasons were identified by Henry Ford for the difficulties with the full management contract program:

> First, the opportunities for contract management within the Greater Detroit area are limited, particularly in light of the serious concerns that many have with the documented excess of beds in the area. In out-state Michigan, the motives of the large, urban hospitals are still viewed with suspicion by many administrators . . . [while] boards of community hospitals are generally unaware of the possibilities or advantages of contractual management. When made aware, community boards, when not faced with an impending crisis, are reluctant to embrace the management influence of an institution such as ours.[31]

As noted earlier, the nature of Henry Ford's medical staff organization may be an issue which arouses opposition among the medical staffs of prospective participants. It is Henry Ford's conclusion, however, that ". . . each successful project conducted in hospitals of more limited resources helps to dispel the suspicion and reluctance."[32]

That considerable effort will be necessary to "dispel the suspicion and reluctance" is evidenced by Henry Ford's experience with River District Hospital. In the words of one observer, ". . . the hospital is definitely benefiting by the availability of the services that Ford is making available . . ."[33] However, River District has resisted the development of a more formal relationship which would permit the deepening and expansion of cooperative services between the two institutions. Again, it is Henry Ford's conclusion that their ". . . apprehension derives from a strong sense of independence, some suspicion of the motives of a large, urban medical center, and a perceived threat to security on the part of River District supervisory staff."[34]

Despite these early difficulties in some areas, in a recent and highly significant development, Henry Ford's efforts in the area of full management contracts finally bore fruit with the signing of a contract in December 1978 to manage a prepaid health plan in Detroit. The plan, to be known as the Health Alliance Plan, will serve to link the former Metropolitan Health Plan, a prepaid group practice comprised of two plan hospitals and five plan "health centers" in the Greater Detroit area, to the Henry Ford Hospital system. Metropolitan Health Plan subscribers and providers will be retained under the new management.

The specifics of the contract conform closely to the model contract outlined earlier. An administrator has been hired as an employee of Henry Ford with the approval of the Plan board to whom the administrator reports and who retain the right of terminating the administrator should events so dictate. The fee for the three year contract is based upon an estimation of costs. As in the other management service arrangements, special consultative services from staff of Henry Ford Hospital are available on a fee basis.[35]

During the grant period, there was substantial activity in short-term specific assistance. As a result, new resources and skilled manpower were applied to previously neglected or inadequately addressed problems, leading to improvement in both the management and clinical aspects of the delivery of services for a number of institutions. The relationship with River District Hospital clearly has benefited that institution, and the activities of Consolidated Hospital Resources represent a promising forum for joint efforts.

The financial aspects of the Institutional Services Program showed positive results. Higher than expected activity levels from short-term consultation services led to significantly higher service generated revenues than anticipated while expenses also increased but to a proportionately lesser extent.[36] The Henry Ford commitment to continue the Institutional Services Program following the end of grant support further points to the financial viability of the program.

The reaction to the Institutional Services Program by Henry Ford management and professional staff was reported to be one of enthusiasm deriving from the enjoyment of ". . . sharing background(s) and talents with others."[37] The medical staff's active participation in the development and implementation of continuing medical education and other clinically related projects is evidence of support of the Institutional Services Program by this important constituency. Indeed, the numerous requests for continuing medical education programs by medical staffs throughout the state point to this type of activity as an important tool in introducing hospitals and medical staffs to multi-institutional arrangements and the opportunities for further affiliation. Henry Ford identified the "nonthreatening nature and the continuing emphasis of accrediting and licensing bodies" as two important factors that lead to the high level of activity and acceptance of educational programs, be they related to medical or nonmedical personnel and subject matter.[38]

On balance, it would seem that the Henry Ford system, by making available clinical and management resources and by working in conjunction with other area institutions, offers a promising development in interorganizational arrangements. Further, the recent management contract signed with a prepaid group practice, the already existing suburban satellite clinics, and the several programs designed to serve inner city residents suggests substantial progress towards a system integrated not only horizontally but vertically as well.

REFERENCES

1. Brown, Montague and Lewis, Howard L. *Hospital Management Systems: Multi-Unit Organization and Delivery of Health Care*, Germantown, MD: Aspen Systems Corporation, 1976.
2. Henry Ford Hospital. "Proposal for Support to Initiate a Program for the Development and Improvement of a Health Care System." Grant proposal submitted to the W. K. Kellogg Foundation, October 10, 1974.
3. Ibid.
4. Ibid.
5. Henry Ford Hospital. "Draft of Proposal to Initiate a Program for the Development and Improvement of a Health Care System." Submitted to W. K. Kellogg Foundation.
6. Klicka, Karl S., M.D. "Field Notes: Henry Ford Hospital, Detroit, Michigan, February 22, 1977." Report to the W. K. Kellogg Foundation.
7. Henry Ford Hospital. "Proposal for Support to Initiate a Program . . ."
8. DeVries, Robert A. "Development of a Health Care System: Henry Ford Hospital." *Program Notes:* W. K. Kellogg Foundation, 1974.
9. Henry Ford Hospital. "Proposal for Support to Initiate a Program . . ."
10. DeVries, "Development of a Health Care System: Henry Ford Hospital . . ."
11. Henry Ford Hospital. "Annual Report, Institutional Services Program, Henry Ford Hospital." Submitted to the W. K. Kellogg Foundation, January 31, 1977.
12. Henry Ford Hospital. "Annual Report, Institutional Services Program, Henry Ford Hospital." Submitted to the W. K. Kellogg Foundation, January 31, 1976.
13. Henry Ford Hospital. "Annual Report . . ." 1977.
14. Henry Ford Hospital. "Annual Report . . ." 1976.
15. Henry Ford Hospital. "Annual Report . . ." 1977.
16. Henry Ford Hospital. "Annual Report . . ." 1976.
17. Henry Ford Hospital. "Annual Report . . ." 1977.
18. Henry Ford Hospital. "Annual Report . . ." 1976.
19. Henry Ford Hospital. "Annual Report . . ." 1977.
20. Henry Ford Hospital. "Annual Report . . ." 1976.
21. Henry Ford Hospital. "Annual Report, Institutional Services Program, Henry Ford Hospital." Submitted to the W. K. Kellogg Foundation, January 31, 1978.
22. Henry Ford Hospital. "Annual Report . . ." 1977.
23. Henry Ford Hospital. "Annual Report . . ." 1976.
24. Henry Ford Hospital. "Annual Report . . ." 1978.
25. Henry Ford Hospital. "Annual Report . . ." 1977.
26. Ibid.
27. Henry Ford Hospital. "Annual Report . . ." 1978.
28. Ibid.
29. Klicka, "Field Notes: Henry Ford Hospital. . ."
30. Brown and Lewis, *Hospital Management Systems* . . .
31. Henry Ford Hospital. "Annual Report . . ." 1977.

32. Ibid.
33. Klicka, "Field Notes: Henry Ford Hospital, . . ."
34. Henry Ford Hospital. "Annual Report . . ." 1978.
35. Telephone conversation with Alan R. Case, Henry Ford Hospital, Detroit, Michigan.
36. Henry Ford Hospital. "Annual Report . . ." 1977.
37. Henry Ford Hospital. "Annual Report . . ." 1976.
38. Henry Ford Hospital. "Annual Report . . ." 1978.

Health Central, Inc.

Background and Structure

Health Central, Inc. is a not-for-profit, multi-unit, health care management and service organization, with corporate offices in Minneapolis, Minnesota. It traces its origins to a loose combination of three suburban Minneapolis hospitals in the mid-sixties. This relationship proved cumbersome in terms of the development and implementation of major business initiatives since each hospital's governing board maintained considerable sovereignty. A decision was made in 1970 to dissolve the existing arrangement and consolidate the organizations into a new corporation, taking the name of the present parent corporation, Health Central, Inc.[1] The late sixties also saw the development of a shared services program by the hospital group in which services were provided to outside independent health care institutions. By the end of 1978, Health Central owned or operated 11 health care facilities with a total capacity exceeding 1,700 beds, and maintained affiliations with more than 100 hospitals and nursing care facilities. Total linkages involved 115 institutions representing more than 10,200 beds in seven upper Midwest states.[2]

In addition to advantages such as lower unit costs, increased ability to attract highly qualified personnel, and better access to capital markets, Health Central President Donald C. Wegmiller sees the chief advantages to such systems in the following context:

> The separation of management into individuals responsible for the direction of the overall system, apart from administrators responsible for the management of individual institutions, has given the health care industry a corporate structure necessary to more effectively plan, finance, and meet the objectives of an organization. The freedom of corporate management to plan, develop, think, and take action on a systemwide basis has proven to be a necessary and positive ingredient for progress.[3]

At Health Central, the corporate structure highlighted in Wegmiller's statement is built around seven owned or operated health care facilities (also known as divisions or member institutions). Three of the institutions (the original three members) are located in suburban Minneapolis: Golden Valley Health Center, Golden Valley; Mercy Medical Center, Coon Rapids; and Unity Hospital, Fridley. Three are located in "outstate" Minnesota: Buffalo Memorial Hospital, Buffalo; St. Mary's Hospital and Home, Winsted; and Long Prairie Memorial Hospital and Home, Long Prairie. The seventh institution is Dakota Midland Hospital in Aberdeen, South Dakota. Another division of the Health Central system is the Health Central Institute, a research and education arm specializing in basic medical research and programs of in-service and community health education.[4]

By the end of 1978, Health Central had expanded its scope to embrace four managed hospitals: Monticello-Big Lake Community Hospital and Home and Granite Falls Municipal Hospital and Manor, both in Minnesota; Ipswich Community Hospital in South Dakota; and Linton Hospital in North Dakota.

Health Central is organized to embrace four areas of governance: ownership, corporate governance, local governance, and management or policy implementation. Health Central's ownership body is known as the Board of Members. It is composed of governing board representation from divisional and member institutions as well as board chairmen of key affiliated hospitals. The Board of Members elects the corporate board of directors and selects corporate auditors.

Corporate governance is provided by an 18 member corporate board of directors drawn from major hospitals in the system and from communities served on an at-large basis. Representatives to this body are nominated by their respective boards of governors and approved by the Health Central corporate board. Duties of the corporate board include: establishing corporate objectives; review and approval of major programming decisions of each division or hospital; appointment and evaluation of the president; appointment of division and hospital governing boards; authorization of borrowing or other major financing; development of long-range planning at the corporate level; review and approval of capital expenditures exceeding $50,000; approval of all contracts; and review and approval of all division and hospital budgets.[5] The third level of governance is provided by boards of governors representing divisions and member institutions. These groups are responsible for: establishment of their individual annual budgets; approval of capital expenditures under $50,000; appointment and evaluation of chief executive officers; development of major hospital objectives, plans, and programs for corporate review; election and appointment of qualified medical staff; evaluation of institutional performance; long range planning at the institutional level; and assurance of high quality health care delivery.[6]

Systemwide management and policy implementation are coordinated through the Office of the President, made up of the President, the Senior Vice President, and the Vice President of Finance. Corporate management staff members coordinate and provide support services in areas such as architectural engineering, biomedical engineering, data processing, finance, planning, public relations, and purchasing.[7]

Divisional and member institutional administrators report to both their local boards and corporate management. For program and policy development, as well as medical staff and community relations, they report to their own divisional boards. For program execution and overall performance, reporting authority lies with the corporate management staff.[8]

Health Central's Shared Services Program offers a wide variety of services to independent institutions under the following broad categories:[9]
- Accounting and Financial Management
- Architectural Engineering
- Management Systems Support
- Biomedical Engineering
- Group Purchasing
- Fund Development
- Ambulance/Emergency Transportation
- In-service and Community Health Education
- General Management Consultation
- Long Range Planning
- Public Relations
- Physician and Personnel Recruitment
- Data Processing
- Interior Design Consultation

Under this program, affiliated institutions pay for services on either a per bed or percentage of salary basis, depending on the service. Of special note is the group purchasing program, described as the largest of its kind in the upper Midwest. Health Central negotiates more than 350 contracts involving over 10,000 supply items for participating institutions. Individual facilities purchase, receive, and are billed for items on a direct basis by vendors, at prices negotiated by Health Central.[10]

From its own experience and from observation of other multi-unit systems, Health Central identified several major obstacles that have been found to interfere with successful consolidations, mergers, and management agreements: (1) a perceived loss of autonomy by the small local hospital; (2) community pride often jeopardized by the need to turn to "the big city" for help; (3) local hospital administrators' apprehension over losing their jobs or image by turning elsewhere for help; (4) anxiety over a perceived need to change the way a hospital does things now in order to adapt to meet the standards of the system; (5) fear by senior physicians that they will lose some of their influence; and (6) the parent corporation's distance from the local hospital and concomitant lack of familiarity with local problems and needs.[11]

In response to these barriers, Health Central developed a strategy that embraced four management contract options under which local hospitals could become part of the system:

1. Corporate Headquarters and Local Facility Option: A more traditional arrangement under which a local hospital receives direct management support from the central organization.
2. Member Hospital and Local Facility Option: Contractual relationship is established between a Health Central hospital and a local health care facility, with back-up support available from the central organization.
3. Shared Services Support Center and Local Facility Option: Health Central affiliates designed as regional support centers, which came to be known as Shared Services Support Centers, would contract for full management services with a local health facility.
4. Affiliated Hospital and Local Facility Option: Management contract relationships would be established between a hospital or other health care facility affiliated with Health Central under the shared services program, and the local health care facility.

The system structure thus involved a complex network of relationships allowing outside institutions to attach themselves to the system (via management contract in this particular instance, but also through various levels of participation ranging in commitment from ownership to affiliation through shared services) at four different points in the network. This structure is seen as an innovative way of fostering system growth while mitigating against the fears and anxieties that often accompany and may prevent management contract agreements.

The Shared Services Support Center (SSSC) is a mechanism by which Health Central implements its shared services program in several large sectors of its service region. Health Central's experience showed that certain shared services, such as management assistance and data processing, could be more efficiently and economically dispensed through decentralized support institutions rather than through one central office. Hence, there arose affiliation agreements with, in most instances, independent health care facilities meeting certain criteria, under which Health Central renders shared services to them while they in turn serve as SSSCs, offering shared services to other neighboring small health care facilities. Several criteria were developed whereby an institution could be designated as a Shared Services Support Center: the support center hospital should be a 150-200 bed hospital (although they need not necessarily be hospital-based) under a nonprofit corporation; the institution should represent a community recognized as an area economic center; the institution should have the capacity to serve institutions up to 100 miles distant; and the institution should express a willingness to serve and develop working relationships with smaller neighboring institutions.[12]

Three SSSC models were envisioned. In the first, the "facility focus" or "inhouse" model, the Health Central Director of Shared Services would relate to a support center coordinator who would be a member of the affiliated hospital's administrative staff. In turn, the coordinator would relate to the neighboring facilities. The second model, the "storefront" model, would be characterized by offices maintained apart from the affiliated health facility and would provide services such as printing and warehousing which require separate facilities. The support center may even carry a different name from the hospital with which it is tied. The third model, the "territory" model, has a single coordinator responsible for two or more support centers, an arrangement felt to be particularly appropriate in service areas with small population bases.[13]

In 1978, Health Central approached the W. K. Kellogg Foundation with a proposal for funding the development of the four management services options. The Foundation agreed to provide assistance amounting to $319,150 on a declining basis for a three year period. The grant was to be supplemented by projected management fees of approximately $448,000 and an in-kind contribution of $75,000 from Health Central bringing the total funds for development of management contracts to over $842,000 over three years.[14] The Kellogg grant focused on the latter three management contract options which emphasized management contract through decentralized units of the Health Central system. Five project goals were identified for the funding period:[15]

1. Establish at least six contractual relationships for general management services between local hospitals associated with Health Central.
2. Establish organizational environments within the managed hospitals conducive to the ongoing strengthening of the relationships between their operations and the managing facilities.
3. Improve the managing organization's capabilities in the areas of management and clinical support to its managed facilities and to neighboring health care facilities.
4. Evaluate the advantages accruing to hospitals which participate with a multi-unit system via management contract support within the varied models.
5. Share the results of the demonstration project with other hospitals and hospital systems throughout the United States.

From this development program arose a management relationship between Dakota Midland Hospital, Health Central's member institution in Aberdeen, South Dakota, and Ipswich Community Hospital, a 19 bed hospital in a community of 1,200 located 30 miles from Aberdeen. As a Health Central shared services affiliate, the Ipswich hospital had developed a two year working relationship with Dakota Midland. This paved the way for ensuing discussions with administrators of the larger, neighboring hospital centering on Ipswich management concerns. The agreement was effected in January 1978.

Although Dakota Midland is designated as a SSSC (Aberdeen Shared Services Support Center) these relationships are categorized under the member hospital and local facility option, Dakota Midland being one of Health Central's member hospitals.

Terms of the contract specify an initial agreement for a period of one year unless sooner terminated upon 60 day notice by either party. Upon expiration of the first year, the agreement shall automatically renew itself for each of the two successive years unless 30 days prior to the beginning of the second year the managed hospital's board informs the managing hospital otherwise in writing.[16]

The Dakota Midland/Ipswich Community agreement includes three general categories, or packages, of services. Under the basic services package, Dakota Midland recommends to the Ipswich board for their approval an administrator for Ipswich who will be carried on the Dakota Midland payroll, report to the Ipswich board and be responsible to the Dakota Midland administrator. The basic package also makes available to Ipswich the following personnel from Dakota Midland: Comptroller, Coordinator of Shared Services, Director of Materials Management, Supervisor of Medical Records, Director of Public Information, Director of Food Services, Dietitian, Director of Nursing Services, Director of Pharmacy Services, Housekeeping Supervisor, Cardiopulmonary Supervisor, Social Services Coordinator, and Volunteer Coordinator.

The second package furnishes general management consultation and evaluation services of the Dakota Midland Administrator and the Health Central President, Senior Vice President, and Shared Services Director. The third package includes all other consulting and support services listed earlier under Health Central's shared services program.[17]

The fee structure is tied to the benefit packages. An annual fee covers the basic service package, including the administrator's salary, the general management and evaluation package, and other consulting services. Additional consulting services, available on an hourly basis of one and one-half times the consultant's hourly wage, must be approved by the local board.[18]

Several other aspects of the contract are notable: Dakota Midland and Health Central are freed from all liability for debts or losses incurred by Ipswich Community, Dakota Midland is covered on all Ipswich insurance policies, and all contracts with physician specialists and Blue Cross are in no way affected.[19]

With respect to the power and authority of the Ipswich governing board, the agreement includes a clause which reads as follows:

> Nothing in this agreement is intended to alter or displace the authority and responsibility of the Board of Trustees of Ipswich Community Hospital. The Board of Trustees shall retain full responsibility in terms of management, control, and policy decisions with such responsibility to be exercised according to those fiduciary obligations customarily residing with such a board.[20]

In March 1978, the 34 bed hospital and 122 bed nursing home at Long Prairie, Minnesota, 200 miles from Minneapolis, was linked to Health Central under a lease-purchase agreement similar to those under which other Health Central member institutions became involved with the organization. For practical purposes, however, this arrangement can be better characterized as a management contract under the Corporate Headquarters and Local Facility Option.[21]

Under the agreement the Long Prairie City Council was relieved of management responsibility for the hospital, home, and adjacent medical clinic. The institution's board of governors retained full policy making authority, full trusteeship of all properties, and responsibility for selection and appointment of qualified medical staff. The Long Prairie administrator reports directly to the local board of governors and retains full management authority with management support from Health Central as required, and Health Central assumes ultimate financial and operational responsibility for a term of 20 years guaranteeing payment of all principal and interest on outstanding bonds of the hospital, home, and clinic during that period.

Later in 1978, Monticello-Big Lake Community Hospital, serving communities just west of the Minneapolis metropolitan area, entered a traditional management contract with Health Central. At almost the same time, another management contract, based on the Corporate Headquarters and Local Facility Option, was effected with Granite Falls Municipal Hospital and Manor, serving a community of 3,500 in western Minnesota. In both cases, ratification of the agreement was predicated upon Health Central's recruitment of a new administrator for the facility and subsequent approval by the board.[22]

In late 1978, there was concluded a second decentralized management contract under the Member Hospital and Local Facility Option wherein trustees of Lincoln Hospital, serving Linton, North Dakota, voted to contract with Dakota Midland Hospital for management services. Under this three year agreement, Linton Hospital receives the three service packages identified under the Ipswich/Dakota Midland model.[23]

Implementation and Process

Health Central developed a detailed project methodology to guide the implementation of the management contract relationship. At the corporate level, initial steps call for the development of criteria for the selection of managed and managing hospitals from which a list of prime candidates for both roles is developed. Corporate staff then visit with potential candidates, detailing the proposed management contract arrangement to the institutions' boards and administrative personnel. As more contracts are established, Health Central is developing a "cadre" of trustees, medical staff, and department heads, knowledgeable about the various aspects of management contracts, who will assist in these presentations by educating their counterparts in potential contracting institutions as to the benefits arising from such relationships.[24]

At the managed institution level, once a contract has been signed the first step calls for a broad orientation for all leading participants in the organization. At Ipswich Community, the process of orientation and continued monitoring of the progress of the contract by the Ipswich board is accomplished in several ways. The administrator of Ipswich attends governing board meetings at Dakota Midland, reporting on the progress and developments of the relationship. Likewise, the Dakota Midland administrator attends meetings of the Ipswich board. The two boards also meet together on a periodic basis. Members of both boards jointly attend various educational seminars sponsored by Health Central and other organizations.[25]

The managed institution's administrator also participates in a series of orientation meetings with the managing institution's administration in which a review of all matters of mutual concern are addressed: strengths and weaknesses in the management of both institutions; strategies for improvement; the range of available contract services; opportunities for developing further shared relationships with other neighboring institutions; and the potential for development of middle management staff.[26] Under the Ipswich/Dakota Memorial agreement, the administrator of Ipswich serves as the coordinator of the Dakota Midland Shared Services Center program in addition to his Ipswich administrative responsibilities. His orientation began at Health Central headquarters in Minneapolis. Serving under the immediate supervision of the Dakota Midland administrator, he enjoys close consulting relationships with the entire Dakota Midland management staff, attends Dakota Midland management council meetings, and has direct access to Health Central corporate staff with whom he meets on a monthly basis.[27]

Orientation of department heads takes place in joint meetings of department head staffs representing managed and managing institutions where the nature of the contract relationship is outlined and opportunities for the sharing of expertise and resources are appraised.[28] Plans for in-service education programs at Ipswich, utilizing Dakota Midland staff in physical therapy, inpatient education, respiratory therapy, and nursing services, are the first areas to develop the sharing potential by these middle management groups.[29]

Public orientation efforts are aimed at reducing anxieties that often accompany significant changes in the operation of a community hospital, and at encouraging future positive involvement by the community in charting the course of the institution.[30] At Ipswich, the governing board held a public meeting prior to instituting the agreement with Dakota Midland at which the proposed contract was explained and discussed.

The hospital's annual meeting provided another forum at which the elements of the relationship were explained.[31]

The Health Central implementation strategy next calls for an analysis of past accounting and budgeting practices and related financial statements, followed by the development of strengthened fiscal procedures compatible with the managing institution's systems.[32] At Ipswich, this review was performed by the Dakota Midland comptroller in conjunction with the Ipswich administrator and revealed obsolete and redundant manual accounting practices and a management information system that was difficult to utilize. Initial corrective steps involved reorganization of Ipswich fiscal systems in preparation for "interfacing" them with the Dakota Midland computer.[33]

An important step in the Health Central implementation strategy deals with long range planning development in managed institutions. This part of the strategy calls for particularly heavy involvement by Health Central corporate staff. In addition, mechanisms are established to insure participation by administration, governing board, medical staff, and community leadership. A four stage process is outlined:[34]

1. Conduct analysis of participating organizations' service to identify service needs and resources . . .
2. Develop policy and procedures for long-range planning . . .
3. Conduct orientation sessions in long-range planning for trustees, medical staff, and department staffs . . .
4. Prepare preliminary draft of a three year role and program plan for the managed hospital and its relationship to the managing organization and/or Health Central, Inc. . . .

At Ipswich, this process centers around a long-range planning committee made up of three Ipswich board members, the president of the Ipswich auxiliary, the Ipswich administrator, the administrator of an Ipswich nursing home, and citizen representatives from two neighboring communities. The committee has thus far operated through the review of a series of "issue papers" which furnish the basis for deliberation over matters such as available clinical services in Ipswich, Ipswich physical facilities, and shared services opportunities.[35]

In pursuit of the third goal of the program (i.e., improve the managing organization's capabilities in the areas of management and clinical support to its managed facility and to neighboring health care facilities) several tasks are identified. The first calls for an assessment of capabilities and needs of the managing organization with an eye towards identifying services with potential to be shared with other organizations.

A second task involves the integration of managed facilities into the central purchasing program and consultative services offered by managing facilities and Health Central. Both steps call for active participation by Health Central corporate staff.[36]

A final step in the implementation process calls for evaluation by all participants of the performance and benefits accruing to institutions affected by the program. Plans call for the evaluation to consider subjective information, such as attitudes of governing boards, medical staffs, department heads, and the general public, and objective data such as service utilization profiles, costs per admission and patient day, percentage increases in patient revenues and expenses, and financial savings from the shared purchasing program and other related services.[37]

Impact and Outcome

Thus far, there are signs that the structure and implementation process designed by Health Central are promising.

Several early indications from Ipswich point to success in overcoming the initial fears identified earlier as barriers to successful operation under management contract arrangements. For example, the Ipswich administrator has reported:[38]

> The boards of the two hospitals are increasingly enthusiastic over the success of their joint venture . . . The Ipswich board is very pleased with the support in long range planning, the development of shared services, and with how responsive Dakota Midland has been to Ipswich Community Hospital's needs.
> The medical staff at Ipswich has remained unaffected by the agreement. The contract has not influenced referral patterns nor affected the patient/physician relationships.
> The local leadership and pride in the hospital has been enhanced by this relationship and by the success that the board has encountered in dealing with issues that previously seemed beyond the capability of the hosptial.

In the short time period that the contract has been in effect, a net cost savings after the contract fee of $28,644 has been realized from the switch to Dakota Midland's data processing system (savings in employee salaries), from the group purchasing plan, and in the administrator's salary.[39] The potential for savings in other institutions is evidenced by a study performed by Health Central in which purchasing systems of 23 other institutions were audited. A combined savings of $600,000 per year was identified as representing savings which could have been effected had the audited institution participated in Health Central's group purchasing program.[40]

The growth of Health Central, evidenced by the increase in agreements reached with other institutions, would indicate the organization's ability to demonstrate and provide beneficial service to those electing to participate.

Currently, Health Central is considering the establishment of two decentralized management agreements under the support center and local facility option.[41] The first proposal would link two Health Central affiliates–St. Michael's Hospital, Tyndall, South Dakota and St. Benedict Hospital, Parkston, South Dakota–to Sacred Heart Hospital, which houses Health Central's Lewis and Clark SSSC in Yankton, South Dakota, under a management contract. Sacred Heart, a 200 bed institution, would provide a single administrator to oversee both of the institutions.

Sacred Heart, as the prime manager, would provide a broad scope of services to the managed hospitals at the department head level. As co-manager, Health Central will provide additional support services as outlined in its other decentralized management involvements.

A refinement of the support center/local facility option is characterized by a proposal linking Health Central to a separate nonprofit corporation which would become prime manager of four institutions serving contiguous areas in north central Minnesota. In this proposal, the administrator of Douglas County Hospital, currently a Health Central SSSC in Alexandria, Minnesota, would become chief executive officer of Lakes Area Health Services, a new organization which would provide management services to smaller area hospitals under contract. Hospitals served under the arrangement would be represented on the regional organization's board in order to preserve local control. Health Central would supply support services to the regional organization under contract.

One of the hospitals to be served is the 34 bed Memorial Hospital of Long Prairie, Minnesota, discussed earlier as already a member institution under a lease-purchase agreement. The others are Douglas County Hospital, 101 beds; Minnewaska District Hospital, 19 beds, Starbuck, Minnesota; and Stevens County Memorial Hospital, 48 beds, Morris, Minnesota.

In addition, Health Central is engaged in and planning to develop several other programs exhibiting elements of both vertical and horizontal integration. Corporate management has assisted in the development of four medical office buldings under a variety of ownership, operational, and affiliative arrangements.[42] Health Central was the force behind the development of a "captive offshore" insurance company presently meeting the malpractice insurance needs of member hospitals. There are plans to explore further the company's role in meeting other hospital insurance requirements.[43] Future plans also call for the development of ambulatory care programs via hospital-based and free-standing models.[44]

Thus, to this point, Health Central is a system marked by growth and activity in a variety of areas, with indications of exploration of new avenues of organizational integration.

REFERENCES

1. Wegmiller, Donald C. "From a Hospital to a Health Care System: A Case Example." *Health Care Management Review*, 3:61-67, Winter 1978.
2. Gehant, David P. "Preliminary Report: Establishing 'Regional Support Centers' to Decentralize Shared Service Programs and Management Support in a Multi-Unit Organization." Report to the Kellogg Foundation and the Hospital Research and Educational Trust, October 12, 1978.
3. Wegmiller, "From a Hospital . . ."
4. Gehant, "Preliminary Report: Establishing 'Regional Support Centers' . . ."
5. Wegmiller, "From a Hospital . . ."
6. Ibid.
7. Ibid.
8. Ibid.
9. Gehant, "Preliminary Report: Establishing 'Regional Support Centers' . . ."
10. Wegmiller, "From a Hospital . . ."
11. "Alternate Contractual Relationships for Local Hospitals to Join a Multi-Unit Hospital Organization." Submitted by Health Central, Inc. to the W. K. Kellogg Foundation, 1978.
12. Wegmiller, Donald C. "Multi-Institutional Pacts Offer Rural Hospitals Do-or-Die Option." *Hospitals, J.A.H.A.*, 52:51-54, January 16, 1978.
13. Gehant, "Preliminary Report: Establishing 'Regional Support Centers' . . ."
14. DeVries, Robert A. "Rural Multi-Hospital Management, Health Central, Inc." *Program Notes:* W. K. Kellogg Foundation, 1978.
15. "Alternate Contractual Relationships for Local Hospitals to Join a Multi-Unit Hospital Organization . . ."
16. Gehant, "Preliminary Report: Establishing 'Regional Support Centers' . . ."
17. Ibid.
18. Gehant, "Preliminary Report: Establishing 'Regional Support Centers' . . ."
19. Ibid.
20. Ibid.
21. "Alternate Contractual Relationships for Local Hospitals to Join a Multi-Unit Hospital Organization . . ."
22. Personal communication from James F. Moffet, Health Central, Inc., March 14, 1979.
23. Ibid.
24. "Alternate Contractual Relationships for Local Hospitals to Join a Multi-Unit Hospital Organization . . ."
25. Ibid.
26. Ibid.
27. Gehant, "Preliminary Report: Establishing 'Regional Support Centers' . . ."
28. "Alternate Contractual Relationships for Local Hospitals to Join a Multi-Unit Hospital Organization . . ."

29. Gehant, "Preliminary Report: Establishing 'Regional Support Centers' . . ."

30. "Alternate Contractual Relationships for Local Hospitals to Join a Multi-Unit Hospital Organization . . ."

31. Gehant, "Preliminary Report: Establishing 'Regional Support Centers' . . ."

32. "Alternate Contractual Relationships for Local Hospitals to Join a Multi-Unit Hospital Organization . . ."

33. Gehant, "Preliminary Report: Establishing 'Regional Support Centers' . . ."

34. "Alternate Contractual Relationships for Local Hospitals to Join a Multi-Unit Hospital Organization . . ."

35. Ibid.

36. Ibid.

37. Ibid.

38. Gehant, "Preliminary Report: Establishing 'Regional Support Centers' . . ."

39. Ibid.

40. Wegmiller, "Multi-Institutional Pacts . . ."

41. Personal communication, James A. Moffet, March 14, 1979.

42. Wegmiller, "From a Hospital . . ."

43. Ibid.

44. Ibid.

Nebraska Methodist Hospital— Shared Services Systems

Background and Structure

In less than 10 years, Nebraska Methodist Hospital has expanded multi-institutional arrangements from a shared laundry, serving two facilities, to shared services for 60 institutions and six management contracts in three states. Nebraska Methodist, a 606 bed general hospital, has achieved this growth in multi-unit services through Shared Services Systems, a totally owned operating division of Nebraska Methodist. The origins of Shared Services Systems can be traced to 1968 when Nebraska Methodist moved into a newly constructed facility, converting the old building into a long-term care center for the chronically ill, the Eugene C. Eppley Complex. The Eppley Complex provided laundry and certain central supply services for Nebraska Methodist, in return obtaining supply and purchasing services.

In the years immediately following, a series of events provided Nebraska Methodist with the impetus for further development of shared services and entry into other multi-unit arrangements. The existing sharing agreement, recognized by the participants as having the potential to yield savings through economies of scale, was being hampered by the obsolescence of the Eppley laundry. Nebraska Methodist wished to convert space then utilized for supply storage to other uses. At the same time, other area health institutions were beginning to indicate interest in participating in the arrangement. Subsequently, Nebraska Methodist purchased a large existing structure and converted it to house the Shared Services Systems operations. In addition, Nebraska Methodist had hired a consulting group to assist them in the formulation of a long range plan. The consulting study discouraged physical expansion through the addition of more beds to existing facilities, recommending instead organizational expansion through management agreements ". . . as a means to maintain and expand a competent staff of managerial and professional personnel."[1] This recommendation coincided with a desire on the part of the Board of Nebraska Methodist to assist other health care facilities to cope with an increasingly complex managerial and health care delivery environment.

The full management without ownership model was seen by Shared Services Systems as a particularly appropriate mechanism for rural hospitals where problems of access to care and financial instability are particularly severe. Despite these difficulties, the service that rural hospitals provide to their communities was seen as vital by Shared Services Systems. These hospitals are the first stop for the victim of an auto accident on Interstate 80 and often the only skilled help available for the farmer injured on the job. The objective of the Shared Services Systems program was to strengthen these ". . . front line health care institutions in the agricultural belt of mid-America . . . through the injection of the correct mixture of personnel and systems to allow the institution to re main under local control and continue its health care mission unimpeded."[2]

The first management contract was signed in 1971 with Children's Memorial Hospital, a 100 bed nonprofit pediatric hospital in Omaha. The situation at Children's was, in many respects, representative of that found in other hospitals which later entered the system. The hospital had been without an administrator for five months and was experiencing a $250,000 annual operating loss which was being subsidized by gifts to the hospital.[3] Subsequent contracts were entered with hospitals in the agricultural areas of Nebraska, Iowa, and Missouri within a 150 mile radius of Omaha. These hospitals ranged in size from 29 to 80 beds, and were located in communities with as few as 800 population. Shared Services Systems identified the following as problems which commonly characterize the contract hospitals:[4]

- Severe cash flow problems, compounded by poor accounts receivable turnover
- Poor business and auditing practices
- Little participation by medical staffs in medical audit and utilization review

- Numerous Medicare survey deficiencies
- No long-range planning
- Poorly defined job descriptions and wage/salary programs
- Overstaffing
- Little community involvement
- Uninformed governing boards
- Lack of administrative leadership
- Weak department heads

The response at Children's Hospital was a full management contract whereby Nebraska Methodist furnished an administrator who was responsible to the Board of Children's Hospital while remaining an employee of Nebraska Methodist. Top level management personnel of Nebraska Methodist were made available for consultation at the discretion of the new administrator. Services of hourly Nebraska Methodist personnel were offered at a fee based upon a multiple of their hourly wage. Previously existing agreements of Children's Hospital were to be honored and the governing board maintained its traditional autonomous role.[5] This agreement became the basic model for other management contracts. The inhouse administrator reports both to the Executive Director of Shared Services Systems and to the governing board of the contracting hospital. The administrative and clinical consulting services are available to contracting and noncontracting institutions alike, as are the linen, purchasing, and supply services of Shared Services Systems.

In some instances, a more flexible approach to the structure of the management contract agreement is required. For example, in response to an unusually sensitive situation, a different type of agreement, called a "directed administrative agreement," was developed. In this particular case, an investigation uncovered extensive problems among the administration, medical staff, and community. The situation was so tense that the governing board had considered closing the hospital, even though they were in the process of constructing a new addition. The final agreement that was negotiated placed an administrator, on leave of absence from Shared Services Systems, on the payroll of the local hospital. The Executive Director of Shared Services Systems agreed to act as a special consultant to the governing board and to supervise the work of the newly placed administrator. The agreement was also subject to cancellation by either party upon thirty day notice, without penalty to either party.[6] In this situation, the arrangement allowed the hospital to secure many of the benefits of the basic model without having to make the more extensive commitment.

In 1974, the Executive Director of Shared Services Systems assumed the responsibility for management contracts. A six member committee of the Nebraska Methodist board oversees the policies and programs of Shared Services Systems. This committee meets regularly with the Executive Director of Shared Services Systems and reports on approved programs and management agreement recommendations to the entire Nebraska Methodist board.

By 1976, Shared Services Systems had entered into three management contracts: Children's Memorial Hospital, Fairfax Community Hospital, Fairfax, Missouri; and Plainview Public Hospital, Plainview, Nebraska. Shared Services Systems was concerned, however, that other institutions which could benefit from management contracts were also those least able to afford the dollar commitment necessary to explore and enter into a contract. Thus, Shared Services Systems turned to the W. K. Kellogg Foundation, which responded with a grant for $267,000 over a three year period on a declining basis. The grant was designed to cover the cost of feasibility studies and to offset some of the start up costs of the resulting management contracts and consulting services. A target of nine hospitals under contract by the end of the period was established. The remainder of the program was to be supported by income generated from service fees (approximately 60 percent of anticipated costs) with a goal of financial self-sufficiency by the end of the grant period.[7]

Implementation and Process

Shared Services Systems has adopted an active but restrained marketing strategy for its management contract program. Its intent is to give the program high visibility in hopes of attracting potential clients rather that directly soliciting health care facilities. Although inquiries have been made by incumbent administrators, Shared Services Systems, as a matter of policy, will enter discussions concerning management contracts only if initiated by the governing board of a hospital in which the administrator's position is vacant.[8]

The marketing process began with an inventory of all nonprofit health care facilities within 150 miles of Omaha. The inventory includes such information as size, location, operating statistics, and governing board composition. Publicity is provided through several media, including brochures distributed to consultants, state hospital associations, state medical societies, and state health departments. Special attention is given to educating the medical staffs of institutions already under contract concerning the arrangements in the hope that they will communicate the concept to referral physicians practicing in other hospitals. Educational forums introducing trustees and administrators to the program are also conducted. In 1978, the marketing effort came under the direction of a new marketing division established by Nebraska Methodist to serve both Shared Services Systems and Nebraska Methodist in their various endeavors.[9]

Once contact by a governing board has been made, the first step in implementing a management contract is an extensive feasibility study. Although the study focuses on financial management, nursing, and the medical staff, many other facets of hospital operations also are investigated.[10] The feasibility study conducted for the Tilden Community Hospital in Tilden, Nebraska is typical of the process used. In March 1976, the president of the governing board of Tilden Community contacted the Executive Director of Shared Services Systems to request that the feasibility of a management contract be explored. This 29 bed hospital had been without an administrator for several months. The study involved nine resource people supplied by Nebraska Methodist who examined wage and salary programs, auditor's findings, Medicare and life safety inspection reports, hospital policies, laboratory and radiology service agreements, and medical audits. Additionally, documents of incorporation, corporate and medical staff bylaws, and board minutes were reviewed. A survey was conducted to assess attitudes of the community towards the hospital. Throughout the study, interviews were conducted with members of the governing board, medical staff, departmental personnel, and community leaders.

Based on the feasibility study, a recommendation as to affiliation is made to the governing board of Nebraska Methodist. In most cases a contract is recommended. The study committee has, on occasion, concluded that a particular hospital could not benefit from a management contract at that particular time, while in other cases a determination has been made that an institution is healthy enough to proceed on its own. In one extreme case, a short-term financial analysis projected such severe problems that it was felt a change in management would be insufficient to reverse the crisis situation. At this point, the possibility of Nebraska Methodist assuming complete management authority and debt obligations was explored unsuccessfully. Shortly thereafter the hospital went into receivership.

The results of the study also are presented to the governing board and medical staff of the study hospital. Recommendations are often substantial both in number and content. In the Tilden case, for example, 58 recommendations were made. Priority recommendations included the following:[11]

1. Steps to correct the serious financial condition
2. Need for organized physician recruitment
3. Organization of long range planning activities
4. Initiation of a hospital development program
5. Provisions for governing board education
6. Establishment of a comprehensive wage and salary program

Once an agreement has been established, Shared Services Systems provides interim administrative services until a permanent administrator can be placed in the hospital.

In 1975, a six month training program was started to prepare administrators to work in rural hospitals. Trainees are sought from the ranks of college graduates, preferably with a business background, who have indicated an interest in working in a rural setting. Supervised by the Executive Director of Shared Services Systems and the Employee Relations Department of Nebraska Methodist, the program is limited to one trainee at a time who is placed in a hospital as the management contracts are entered. Practical management experience is stressed and the program serves to familiarize the trainee with the resources available and accessible from Nebraska Methodist once the trainee is assigned to a hospital. This practice is designed to assist in bringing the new adminstrator to full effectiveness early in the contract period.

Management communication and continued education are encouraged through quarterly one day meetings of all administrators of managed and managing institutions. Reporting and group discussion takes place along with educational presentations on such topics as physician recruitment, labor relations, and clinic development.

The scope of services provided to the managed hospitals is tailored to meet local needs. Typically, it has been found that substantial consulting support to the administrator is needed at the outset of the management contract. A wide range of consulting assistance is available. The range of specialists utilized and the number of hours required vary according to the situation in each managed institution. In addition to the expected assistance in such administrative areas as finance, data processing, and planning, consultations also take place in patient care related services such as physical therapy, respiratory therapy, and dietetics.

The Nebraska Methodist medical staff has become involved in the program through increased and broadened continuing medical education activities for rural physicians both in contracting and noncontracting hospitals. They have also encouraged medical audit programs and increased involvement by the rural physicians in the Nebraska Methodist Associate Medical Staff.[12]

Impact and Outcome

The impact of the Shared Services Systems management contract program is evidenced in several ways. There are indications, for example, of improvement in the financial health of the contracting institutions. The $250,000 annual operating deficit at Children's Memorial Hospital has been eliminated.[13] Fairfax Community Hospital also began operating "profitably" after entering the contract and, in 1978, was in the process of securing $2.2 million in financing for a combination remodeling and new construction project to remedy Medicare code deficiencies.[14] Tilden Community Hospital eliminated a deficit bank balance and secured $34,000 from intermediaries in back payments and a retroactive per diem increase. Credit and collection policy and procedure revisions cut accounts receivable in half within a year's time.[15]

It would also appear that the capability to provide services to patients has been enhanced. In this regard, the comments of board members and physicians at Tilden Community Hospital are of note. They expressed the opinion that " . . . patient care has been noticeably improved, this in large measure being due to more appropriate staffing and . . . better morale of the personnel."[16] The improved financial situation at Children's Memorial has allowed gifts and endowments formerly used to subsidize operating losses to be applied to initiate new clinical programs such as a genetic counseling program, an expanded poison information center, and an infant transport system.[17] The continuing medical education efforts of the Nebraska Methodist medical staff resulted in more than 300 presentations to rural physicians in the second year of the grant period and Nebraska Methodist was granted the AMA Certificate of Accreditation in Continuing Medical Education, the first institution in the state of Nebraska to achieve such certification.[18] Decreases in the number of Medicare code violations, the initiation of new services, improvements in facilities and equipment, and successful recruitment of new physicians were noted in most of the contracting hospitals.[19]

Evidence of satisfaction by governing boards and other members of the communities is also available. A long range planning survey questionnaire administered by Fairfax Community Hospital to board members, physicians, and community leaders revealed "unanimous approval" of the arrangement.[20] Board members at Tilden Community Hospital called the arrangement " . . . an unqualified success," expressing their opinion that " . . . the management of the hospital had improved dramatically, giving them a sense of security relative to the financial operations of the hospital . . . ."[21] Concrete evidence of community support in Tilden is provided by the $8,000 raised in the first year of a new development program in a community of but 800 people.[22]

Shared Services Systems has found that while the management contract approach has proven favorable, nevertheless there remain many of
the factors that serve to make the operation of small rural hospitals a difficult task. Shared Services Systems has expressed the concern that,
despite the successes achieved to date, there remain long-run problems of
substantial magnitude in many rural communities which must be addressed:

> The size of the hospital, the size and location of the community, and
> the ability to recruit physicians cause these concerns. It has been
> learned that hospitals of 30 beds and under require more manage-
> ment time and concern than do larger hospitals. Simply stated, the
> internal resources are not available and a great deal of external
> assistance is necessary.[23]

To this point, however, both Shared Services Systems and its affiliated
hospitals have generally been satisfied with the arrangement. With the
addition of the Shelby County Myrtue Memorial Hospital in Harlan,
Iowa and the Gentry County Hospital in Albany, Missouri, Shared Services Systems had six hospitals under contract at the midway point of the
grant period. Several feasibility studies were undertaken during that
period and others were anticipated in the final year of the grant, indicating that a market is still available to them, and that their past performance is serving them well in attracting new management agreements.

REFERENCES

1. Picard, William K. Shared Services Systems. Letter and follow-up grant proposal information to Robert A. DeVries, W. K. Kellogg Foundation, March 12, 1976.
2. Picard, William K. Shared Services Systems. Letter and grant proposal to Robert A. DeVries, W. K. Kellogg Foundation , January 28, 1976.
3. Picard, Letter and follow-up grant proposal.
4. Ibid.
5. Ibid.
6. Ibid.
7. DeVries, Robert A. *Program Notes:* W. K. Kellogg Foundation, Spring 1976.
8. Nebraska Methodist Hospital. "Annual Report to the W. K. Kellogg Foundation, 1978."
9. Ibid.
10. Picard, Letter and follow-up grant proposal.
11. Nebraska Methodist Hospital. "Annual Report to the W. K. Kellogg Foundation, 1977."
12. Nebraska Methodist Hospital. "Annual Report . . . 1978."
13. Picard, Letter and follow-up grant proposal.
14. Nebraska Methodist Hospital. "Annual Report . . . 1978."
15. Nebraska Methodist Hospital. "Annual Report . . . 1977."
16. Klicka, Karl S., M.D. "Field Notes: Nebraska Methodist Hospital, Omaha, Nebraska, July 11-13, 1977."
17. Picard, Letter and follow-up grant proposal.
18. Nebraska Methodist Hospital. "Annual Report . . . 1978."
19. Ibid.
20. Picard, Letter and follow-up grant proposal.
21. Klicka, "Field Notes . . . 1977."
22. Nebraska Methodist Hospital. "Annual Report . . . 1977."
23. Ibid.

Presbyterian Hospital Center

Background and Structure

Presbyterian Hospital is the core institution of the Presbyterian Hospital Center, a multi-unit system of health care facilities serving the state of New Mexico. Based in Albuquerque, this nonprofit hospital, governed by a 15 member board appointed by the Synod of the United Presbyterian Church of the United States, is the largest hospital in New Mexico. The 452 bed facility employs over 1,500 people and has over 27,000 admissions per year.[1]

Presbyterian began its multiple hospital activity with the construction in 1970 of a 172 bed satellite facility in Albuquerque, Anna Kaseman Hospital. The impetus behind this move, as related by Presbyterian President Ray Woodham, was to head off the development of a proposed proprietary hospital in the community.[2] However, a discussion of Presbyterian's development of the multi-unit arrangements that ensued immediately thereafter requires first an understanding of the health care environment in New Mexico, seen as the primary determinant of this growth.

There are 44 community general hospitals, with a total of 3,688 beds, scattered throughout New Mexico,[3] a primarily rural state encompassing 122,000 square miles. Most of the hospitals are small–46 percent have less than 50 beds, and only five have more than 200 beds–and are geographically isolated from other health care facilities. The situation of these small rural hospitals is often characterized as of crisis proportions and the early 1970s saw the closing or consolidation of several.[4] At the same time, these rural hospitals are almost always the only primary health care resource in a community. The roots of the problem are seen to lie in the scarcity of physicians and allied health personnel. The Department of Health, Education, and Welfare has declared 28 of New Mexico's 32 counties as physician shortage areas.[5] These problems are compounded by less than adequate financial resources which reflect, in part, the low incomes of the communities in which the hospitals are located: Valencia, Eddy, Lincoln, and Socorro counties, four communities where Presbyterian subsequently became involved, had mean family incomes ranging from a low of $6,360 to a high of $7,870 in 1970.[6] The need for efficient use of scarce resources and the infusion of additional resources required managerial expertise and innovation, as did the increasingly complex technological and regulatory environment.

These forces combined to force several small communities to look to Presbyterian for assistance. Through lease agreements, and in one case an outright purchase, Presbyterian assumed total management control over the following institutions in New Mexico during the period 1971 through 1976:

- The 21 bed Belen General Hospital, Belen
- The 50 bed Artesia General Hospital, Artesia
- The 42 bed Ruidoso-Hondo Valley Hospital, Ruidoso
- The 99 bed Memorial Hospital, Clovis
- The 45 bed Socorro County General Hospital, Socorro

The lease arrangement was chosen as the vehicle for integration for a number of reasons. The institutions which came to Presbyterian typically were in desperate straits, and sought the maximum degree of assistance although, in most cases, did not wish to relinquish ownership (a view shared by Presbyterian). For its part, Presbyterian, recognizing the seriousness of the situations, wished to have sufficient policy and operating control in order to face the critical issues and to make the difficult decisions that would be required. Further, Presbyterian felt that under the circumstances, a long-term commitment was necessary in order to bring about the requisite changes. Also sought was an arrangement whereby Presbyterian could infuse venture capital to the affiliated hospitals.[7]

Substantial efforts have been expended on behalf of these affiliated hospitals, the impetus for which, according to Woodham, lies in a commitment to service by Presbyterian, a commitment which also serves to strengthen his own institution:

We have the advantage, I think, that my organization has of new challenges and in the type of self-renewal and satisfaction you get from doing something new, and doing something in a situation where you are demonstratively reaching out with a helping hand. It sounds corny, but we are helping the hospitals in those communities.[8]

The lease arrangements typically are for ten year periods with an option to renew, except in Clovis where the initial agreement terminated upon completion of a replacement facility, built and owned by Presbyterian under a separate agreement. Presbyterian pays a lease fee of $1, the lease covering all lands, buildings, improvements, and equipment of the hospitals. Presbyterian assumes all insurance and maintenance costs while the lessor assumes the costs of any construction necessary to bring the facility into code compliance. Each hospital is expected to be financially independent, except for Ruidoso where Presbyterian may retain any excess of revenues over expenses. In all other communities such net income must remain in the respective institutions. Some leases are subject to renegotiation after three years at the option of either party or if occupancy falls below 40 percent.[9]

While the hospitals retain ownership under the lease agreements, the Board of Directors of Presbyterian has final authority regarding policies and programs implemented in the affiliate hospitals.[10] Local advisory boards have been established for each affiliate. These boards, which include a representative from the Presbyterian executive staff, meet at least quarterly and make policy recommendations to the Presbyterian board and management. The advisory boards are seen as a mechanism by which the commitment and involvement of the communities in their hospitals can be maintained.[11] In several communities, advisory boards have been active and instrumental in successful physician recruitment efforts.

As the program progressed, it became evident that the managerial needs of the affiliate hospitals were often beyond the capabilities and resources of Presbyterian as the program was then structured.[12] There was also continuing evidence of the need of small rural hospitals as Presbyterian was being approached almost on a weekly basis by community groups and leaders seeking assistance in helping to keep their hospitals open.[13] It was at this point that Presbyterian approached the W. K. Kellogg Foundation for grant assistance to develop a team of trained and experienced professional consultants to supplement the existing Presbyterian central staff in developing and coordinating the implementation of new management techniques and services for existing and potential affiliate hospitals, and for nonaffiliate hospitals as resources permitted. Experience had revealed to Presbyterian that seven areas of hospital operation were in particular need of attention: (1) physician recruitment; (2) dietary department management; (3) professional standards monitoring; (4) nursing consultation, organization, and recruitment; (5) management engineering; (6) continuing education and in-service education; and (7) personnel management.[14] A consulting team comprised of specialists in these areas was hired through the Kellogg grant, which amounted to $350,000 to be distributed on a declining basis over three years, supplemented by contributions from Presbyterian and service revenues of a like amount. The grant agreement established a target of six new affiliations in the three year period. Serving, in effect, as an operating division of Presbyterian, the new "mutual services program" is available not only to the rural affiliates but serves the base hospital in Albuquerque as well. The agreement also established a target of financial self-sufficiency by the end of the third year. The program would then be supported by a direct cost and central expense allocation on a percentage of gross revenue basis, treated as an account payable of the affiliate hospitals, as certain central accounting services were being supported at the time, and by fees generated from services rendered to nonaffiliated institutions.[15]

Direction of the program was placed in the hands of a Project Director whose responsibilities centered around marketing and physician recruitment. The Project Director reports to the Regional Administrator at Presbyterian, as do the administrators of each affiliate hospital. While incumbents are occasionally retained, the affiliate hospital administrators usually are recruited either from within the Presbyterian system or by attracting recent hospital administration program graduates.

Presbyterian's multi-unit activities also extended to a joint venture known as Cooperative Health Services with another major Albuquerque hospital, St. Joseph's Hospital. Formed in 1971 to ". . . pursue solutions to the broad problems of cost and availability of health care in both urban and rural New Mexico through the application of resources from the private sector . . . ,"[16] the cooperative began with shared purchasing between the two hospitals. An HMO sponsored by the 80 physician Lovelace Clinic, in conjunction with the Lovelace-Bataan Medical Center, was seen by both Presbyterian and St. Joseph's as a potential drain on both of their patient loads. As a result, the cooperative then extended into the formation of the New Mexico Health Care Corporation, a nonprofit HMO doing business as "Mastercare, providing comprehensive health services to over 14,000 subscribers."[17] Other programs organized by Cooperative Health Services were: Southwest Health Care Corporation, a nonprofit organization managing five ambulatory care clinics in medically underserved communities; Bernalillo County Health Care Corporation, a nonprofit ambulance service doing business as "Albuquerque Ambulance," and Hospital Home Health Care, an unincorporated nonprofit home health care agency.

Implementation and Process

To this point, indications of interest in the Presbyterian system have been initiated by potential affiliate hospitals. In seeking to determine if an affiliation agreement is feasible, project staff develop a survey of existing area facilities, costs of similar services in the area, social and economic conditions, and population forecasts. Included in the analysis is a long range financial forecast and strategic financial management plan. This information is used in evaluating the program's impact and in focusing the efforts of the project staff.

Basic services such as purchasing, personnel, general accounting, and financial reporting are centralized in Albuquerque. All purchasing of supplies and equipment, including laboratory and pharmacy supplies, is handled at Presbyterian and delivered to the affiliates on a weekly basis. A data processing program written specifically for the affiliates handles all accounts receivable and payable, general ledgers, funds management, payroll, financial statement preparation, and equipment inventory. The affiliates are provided with centralized internal auditing and assistance in budget preparation.

The program activities have focused on the functional specialties around which the project staff was organized, namely physician recruitment, dietary, nursing, management engineering, education, professional standards monitoring, and personnel management. Physician recruitment has been an area of particular emphasis. The Project Director possesses primary responsibility for this area. He has pursued this task by working closely with a variety of groups: the Family Practice Program of the University of New Mexico School of Medicine, the Rural Health Care Committee of the New Mexico Hospital Association, the New Mexico Medical Association, the New Mexico Board of Medical Examiners, and various community groups such as Chambers of Commerce throughout the state.

Another area of considerable activity has been that of developing supplementary management reports focusing on productivity measurement by the management engineering specialists. An approach was developed whereby information already generated could be summarized and compared to productivity standards. The report, which is available to each affiliate twice a month, is somewhat similar to the Hospital Administrative Services, focusing on financial indicators and personnel utilization. Included are the number of full-time equivalents paid per occupied bed, average daily census, total operating expense and income, and income and expense trends. Computerized activity reports are also generated daily showing month to date and year to date collections, and expense and revenue by department. Actual versus budgeted expense by department are generated every pay period. Monthly computer reports of the aging of accounts allows the management of each affiliate to monitor cash flow and business office performance.

Personnel policies and procedures are standardized to the extent possible. Implementation of such systemwide policies is a gradual process and allowances are made recognizing the particular circumstances of each institution. Eventually, all employee benefits such as insurance, pension programs, and vacation policies are to be standardized for employees of all affiliates. Salary schedules have been an area of much study and are established to be competitive in the respective communities. Employee handbooks are prepared for the affiliates reflecting Presbyterian policies.

Presbyterian has set the goal that all affiliates become accredited by the Joint Commission on Accreditation of Hospitals. The professional standards staff consultant has the main responsibility for monitoring these efforts. The consultant works closely with the affiliates' administrative staffs, medical staffs, and department heads in reviewing JCAH and Medicare requirements in determining which areas are not in compliance and working to remedy them. Efforts in most hospitals have been in the areas of revision of medical staff bylaws and organization, safety programs, infection control, department policies and practices, and building code compliance. Mock surveys have been conducted to prepare for JCAH survey-team visits.

Presbyterian feels that one of the most critical factors in maintaining and improving the quality of care in the affiliates has been the absence of adequate numbers of qualified licensed nurses to plan, supervise, and provide needed nursing care.[19] Hence, the staff nursing consultant's activities have focused heavily on recruiting and arranging for substitute coverage in the affiliates. One approach taken to the coverage problem has been the development of "circuit rider nurse staffing" in which a traveling float pool of nurses are available during vacation periods and peak load periods. Considerable effort has also been directed at upgrading nursing care and standardizing nursing care policies. Guidelines are prepared and circulated by the nursing consultant so that local staff may then prepare specific written policies and procedures taking local needs into consideration. The "Nursing Skills" manuals used at Presbyterian have been used as models for emergency room, nursery, labor, and delivery services. Other activities have included nurse specialty preceptorships at Presbyterian in areas such as obstetrics and refresher courses in areas such as coronary care nursing, infection control, and isolation techniques.

The dietary consultant's involvement has included assistance in complying with state and federal regulatory requirements, efficiency evaluations of the respective food services, ongoing training and education of dietary employees, and communication with medical staffs concerning therapeutic diets.[20]

Yet another area of staff specialization is that of educational program development. The educational coordinator has completed educational needs assessments in all affiliates. In addition to the educational programs noted, examples of new educational efforts are seen in rotations at Presbyterian by affiliate clinical laboratory personnel and presentation of in-service workshops by the Presbyterian respiratory therapy department.[21]

A particularly interesting program is the Board Education Project developed by the educational consultant at the request of the Presbyterian Board of Directors Education Committee. The program is aimed at both the Presbyterian board and the affiliated hospitals' advisory boards. The project began in 1978 with a presentation on the goals and mission of the Presbyterian Hospital Center. The team of consultants, created largely through initial Kellogg funding, now is in the process of becoming a permanent part of the Presbyterian organization, and whose activities will be further integrated to serve Albuquerque hospitals as well as the rural affiliates.

Impact and Outcome

Although slightly below anticipated levels, success was achieved in attracting new institutions to the Presbyterian system. The 60 bed McKinley General Hospital in Gallup, New Mexico and the 80 bed Espanola Hospital in Espanola, New Mexico entered into lease agreements in the first and second years of the grant, respectively, while the 58 bed Dr. Dan C. Trigg Memorial Hospital joined the system at the beginning of the third year. The McKinley and Espanola experiences are among the best examples of the program's successes in remedying dire financial situations. One year prior to Presbyterian assuming operational responsibility for McKinley, the hospital lost $350,000. Within a year's time that loss had been reduced to $50,000.[22] The Espanola Hospital was, according to its board chairman, ". . . only a few days from being closed," just prior to the lease agreement. Upon assuming responsibility for the hospital, Presbyterian immediately infused a large amount of operating capital into the operation, thereby enabling it to continue service.[23] Presbyterian's cash resources are available to the affiliates to cope with cash flow problems when they arise, thereby supplementing new financial systems and practices in helping to assure the financial health of the affiliates.[24] It is expected that, over time, Presbyterian will fully recover all funds flowing to the affiliates.[25]

Many discussions were held concerning potential affiliation agreements, indicating that Presbyterian's perception of the market was accurate. Including the agreements entered, 14 institutions from New Mexico, Colorado, and Texas engaged in such discussions in the first two years of the grant period.[26] Activity also increased in the second year of services provided to nonaffiliates.[27]

One of the major successes of the Presbyterian system has been in physician recruitment. Presbyterian has developed a centralized and extensive recruitment program, the results of which have been most encouraging. In the first two and one-half years of the grant period, some 29 physicians in general and specialty practices have located or have indicated the intention of locating in the communities of Artesia, Belen, Espanola, Gallup, Ruidoso, Socorro, and Tucumcari.[28] Another success has been achieved in the recruitment of several Albuquerque specialists for once-a-week or "as-needed" clinics in Belen, Gallup, and Socorro.[29]

The reduction in the number and kind of deficiencies cited by Medicare and JCAH inspectors is another indication of the program's impact on factors related to the quality of patient care. A marked decrease in the number and severity of deficiencies cited in the affiliates has been noted.[30] The professional standards coordinator's role has been of major importance in this regard. In fact, the Department of Health and Social Services, which is the state Medicare certifying agency, has indicated to Presbyterian that the standards coordinator's assistance in the survey process helped to keep open one of the affiliate hospitals that would otherwise have likely been closed for code deficiencies.[31]

The educational programs, only several of which were mentioned, are undoubtedly influential on the capability to provide patient care. Nurse staffing shortages remain a persistent problem, but the over 1,500 hours of traveling float pool registered nurse coverage provided in the second year were of considerable value.[32] Currently, three full-time nurses staff the float pool.

Per diem costs showed an upward trend for the period 1975 through

1976 in all but one affiliate where data were compiled.[33] Although consistent with industrywide trends, the rise is attributed by the Project Director to a cost/quality trade-off, in which Presbyterian has favored quality improvements in the affiliate hospitals.[34] While some cost control measures have been instituted, as seen in McKinley General Hospital where the ratio of FTEs per occupied bed dropped from 5.21 to 3.18 within a year's time following affiliation, the same measure has shown mixed results in other affiliates.[35] On balance, while costs have risen, affiliates have benefited from increased availability of clinical and management personnel, broadened service capability, and improvements in quality.

The reaction from administrators and the advisory boards to the affiliations has been positive. One outside observer related that ". . . each of the administrators in the hospitals . . . testified without reservation to their complete satisfaction . . ."[36] and found as representative the attitude of one advisory board chairman who was ". . . not only positive but enthusiastic in his praise of the services provided to the hospital."[37] These views are encouraging for the future, as suggested by the Project Director's opinion that progress can be made only if the administrators properly understand the role of the program staff and utilize them willingly.[38]

Positive changes within the affiliated hospitals may well depend to a great extent on the reaction of the local medical staffs. A particularly sensitive issue with some physicians has been Presbyterian's efforts in physician recruitment. In one community, the recruitment of a general surgeon was viewed by certain local practitioners as an infringement on their practice.[39] In general, however, it would appear that medical staff support for the Presbyterian system does exist. There is a general recognition that the back-up services from Presbyterian can be of substantial help to the local affiliate. Conversations with several medical staff members, while noting continuing problems such as the nursing shortage, also acknowledge that, in the long run, the hospitals will benefit from affiliation with Presbyterian.[40]

While growth of the Presbyterian system has revolved primarily around hospitals, recent developments suggest a move toward vertical integration. Presbyterian Hospital Center recently received a Health Underserved Rural Area grant from the Department of Health, Education, and Welfare to develop ambulatory rural health programs. The project is aimed at establishing primary care programs integrated with the comprehensive facilities of the Presbyterian Hospital Center. Clinics have been set up and staffed in several communities in Catron County and in

Grants, New Mexico.[41] These recent efforts evidence the continuing evolution of the Presbyterian system as it seeks to address the difficult and complex problems of assuring medical care to residents of rural communities.

REFERENCES

1. Presbyterian Hospital Center. "Proposal to the W. K. Kellogg Foundation: A Rural Health Consortium for New Mexico (A Mutual Services Program for Rural New Mexico Hospitals)." March 12, 1976.
2. Brown, Montague and Lewis, Howard L. *Hospital Management Systems: Multi-Unit Organization and Delivery of Health Care.* Germantown, MD: Aspen Systems Corporation, 1976, p. 214.
3. Presbyterian Hospital Center, "Proposal to the W. K. Kellogg Foundation . . ."
4. Ibid.
5. Ibid.
6. Ibid.
7. Personal communication with Ray Woodham, February 25, 1979.
8. Brown and Lewis, *Hospital Management Systems.*
9. Presbyterian Hospital Center, "Proposal to the W. K. Kellogg Foundation . . ."
10. McMullan, Kevin. Rural Health Consortium, "Site Visit Progress Report: W. K. Kellogg Foundation." Prepared for Karl S. Klicka, M.D., Winter 1977.
11. Brown and Lewis, *Hospital Management Systems.*
12. McMullan, Rural Health Consortium, "Site Visit . . ."
13. Presbyterian Hospital Center, "Proposal to the W. K. Kellogg Foundation . . ."
14. Ibid.
15. McMullan, Kevin. "First Year Annual Report: Rural Health Consortium: Presbyterian Hospital Center." Prepared for the W. K. Kellogg Foundation, June 1977.
16. Presbyterian Hospital Center, "Proposal to the W. K. Kellogg Foundation . . ."
17. Brown and Lewis, *Hospital Management Systems.*
18. Presbyterian Hospital Center, "Proposal to the W. K. Kellogg Foundation . . ."
19. McMullan, Kevin. "Report to the W. K. Kellogg Foundation for the Second Year of a Three-Year Grant." June 1978.
20. McMullan, "First Year Annual Report . . ."
21. McMullan, Kevin. Rural Health Consortium, October 21, 1976. Letter to Robert A. DeVries, W. K. Kellogg Foundation.
22. McMullan, "First Year Annual Report . . ."
23. McMullan, "Report to the W. K. Kellogg Foundation . . ."
24. McMullan, Rural Health Consortium, "Site Visit . . ."
25. Brown and Lewis, *Hospital Management Systems.*
26. McMullan, "First Year Annual Report . . ."
27. McMullan, "Report to the W. K. Kellogg Foundation . . ."
28. Personal communication with Kevin McMullan, February 26, 1979.
29. McMullan, "First Year Annual Report . . ."
30. McMullan, "Report to the W. K. Kellogg Foundation . . ."
31. McMullan, "First Year Annual Report . . ."
32. Klicka, Karl S., M.D. "Field Trip Report: Presbyterian Hospital Center." March 12-15, 1978.

33. McMullan, Rural Health Consortium, "Site Visit . . ."
34. Ibid.
35. Ibid.
36. Klicka, Karl S., M.D. W. K. Kellogg Foundation, "Field Notes: Presbyterian Hospital Center." March 3, 1977.
37. Klicka, "Field Trip Report . . ."
38. McMullan, Rural Health Consortium, "Site Visit . . ."
39. Woodham, Ray and Mondragon, Fred. Presbyterian Hospital Center. Telephone conversation with Robert A. DeVries, W. K. Kellogg Foundation, August 1978.
40. McMullan, "Report to the W. K. Kellogg Foundation . . ."
41. Personal communication with Kevin McMullan, February 26, 1979.

Saginaw General Hospital—
Operation Outreach

Background and Structure

Operation Outreach represents the effort of Saginaw General Hospital, a 405 bed institution located in Saginaw, Michigan, to develop and implement a program through which participating small rural hospitals in Michigan's Thumb Area are provided with full management contract, consultative, and support services. Although possessing several distinctive features, it can generally be categorized as an example of the variant of management contract models distinguished by a single large independent hospital from which services originate or are coordinated.

The program began in 1974 when Saginaw General contracted with Hills and Dales Hospital, a 65 bed hospital in Cass City, Michigan, for the services of an administrator who was then an assistant administrator at Saginaw General and at which he remained an employee.[1] The situation at Hills and Dales prior to the contract agreement in many ways typified that found in the institutions which make up the market for management contracts: a small rural hospital beset by continuing financial difficulties, unable to attract top-notch administrative skill—in fact, Hills and Dales had been without an administrator for over six months—and experiencing low employee morale.[2]

By July 1975, two more Michigan hospitals, the Deckerville Community Hospital, a 22 bed institution, and Harbor Beach Community Hospital, operating 20 beds, had agreed to similar arrangements with

Saginaw General. The Huron Memorial Hospital, a 77 bed hospital in Bad Axe, Michigan was added shortly thereafter.

The central provision of the management contract calls for the contracting hospital to be provided with the services of a full-time administrator who is recruited, hired, employed, paid, and trained by Saginaw General. The hiring of the administrator is subject to the approval of the participating hospital's governing board. The administrator, charged with those duties customarily performed by the chief executive officer of an institution of similar size and characteristics, reports to the Director of Management Services of the Operation Outreach Program of Saginaw General. The Director may serve as the administrator during the training period of an inexperienced executive. Evaluation of the administrator's performance is the joint responsibility of the Director of Management Services and the contracting hospital's governing board. Both the Director of Management Services and the hospital administrator attend the meetings of that governing board and participate without vote. Saginaw General is empowered to replace the administrator at any time, while the contracting governing board may do so upon 30 day notice to Saginaw General during which interim Saginaw General is obligated to provide administrative coverage and to find a permanent replacement within 90 days.[3] In one instance, an arrangement provided for a single administrator to serve two contracting hospitals.[4]

The management contract additionally furnishes the services of other Saginaw General personnel, including the supervisory and coordinating services of the Director of Management Services, a management engineer, and middle management staff, all to the extent deemed appropriate by Saginaw General to fulfill their management responsibilities.

As is common in many management contracts, the contracting hospital's governing board retains all their traditional rights, responsibilities, and authority.[5] Saginaw General's relationship to the participating hospital is essentially that of an independent contractor.[6] With the exception of the administrator, the participating hospital remains the employer of all other personnel. Saginaw General and all its employees are indemnified from any liabilities or judgments against the institution arising out of services provided by the hospital.[7]

The fee arrangement combines a basic annual fixed rate plus a percentage of the budgeted revenues of the contracting hospital. This fee includes the administrator's salary. Any unexpended funds, as determined by a year end audit, are returned to the participating institutions. Termination of the contract is permitted following a 90 day notice by either party.[8]

In addition to the basic service package, participating hospitals also have the option of purchasing the part-time consulting services of other Saginaw General staff. Such services would involve those tasks requiring appreciable time and travel beyond the extent outlined as available in the basic service package. Payment is made on a per diem rate plus mileage and other out-of-pocket expenses. On-site consultations, lengthy document preparation, and time spent conducting conferences on sharing would be representative of such activities.[9]

In an effort to secure additional funds with which to develop new services and extend the implementation of services into additional hospitals, Saginaw General approached the W. K. Kellogg Foundation, which provided grant support amounting to $250,000 of an anticipated $690,000 expense budget over a three year period. The grant proposal detailed the further development of the program planned by Saginaw General. A full-time Director of Operation Outreach was charged with overall responsibility for the program, which in addition to administrative hiring and coordination of service implementation, included marketing and solicitation of new members, contracting for program development work to be done outside of Saginaw General, and subcontracting for services not provided by Saginaw General.[10]

This latter responsibility points to a distinctive aspect of the Operation Outreach program as envisioned in this planning stage and as later implemented in a variety of forms; that is, offering services provided for in the management contract package via subcontractors and, on a fee basis, utilizing expertise available in some of the contracting hospitals to provide services to other contracting, but otherwise unrelated hospitals.

The subcontracting arrangement arose through a relationship that developed between Saginaw General and the Department of Engineering and Operations Research at Wayne State University, several faculty members from which had instituted an annual operating budget development program at the nearby Marlette Community Hospital in 1973. A similar program was instituted at Hills and Dales Community Hospital just prior to the management contract agreement with Saginaw General. At that time, Saginaw General decided that, rather than providing these financial services directly, they would subcontract for these services and management engineering through the nonprofit corporation established by the faculty members, Health Systems Management, Inc., and implement similar programs in the Deckerville and Harbor Beach facilities.[11]

The use of personnel from contracting hospitals for programwide services may be illustrated by an instance in which a nurse from Hills and Dales played the central role in the development and implementation of utilization review and in-service education programs.[12]

The grant assistance provided for service development in four main areas.[13] The first was the development of administrative guide manuals for department heads. Designed to assist the administratively untrained department head, the departmentally tailored manuals were to cover such topics as workload projections, variable staffing, interpretation of periodic accounting reports, and preparation of capital budgets.

The second area addressed what was perceived to be the prohibitively high cost of commercial computer hardware and software leasing programs. Saginaw General proposed to develop software compatible with small affordable computers that hospitals could buy and to provide the technical assistance in adapting software to the needs of the individual hospitals.

The third and fourth areas were in utilization review and educational services. Manuals were to be prepared which outlined procedures for setting up and implementing such programs and for using available expertise and resources from Saginaw General.

The Operation Outreach management contract program was expected to reach feasibility at the level of seven hospitals. Thus, an addition of three to four hospitals by the end of the three year grant period beginning in mid-1976 was set as a target.[14]

Implementation and Process

The programmatic activities implemented can be categorized as administrative support and clinical support. In the administrative support area, the budgeting system arranged through the Wayne State group was instituted in the contracting hospitals. Characterized as a zero-based system, it involved forecasting hospital activity statistics, evaluation of department workload staffing, comparison of productivity measures to local and national standards, and a control loop utilizing monthly departmental cost reports and budgets for "actual vs. budgeted" comparison and analysis.[15]

An exchange-cart system was instituted in contracting institutions.[16] This materials management system was seen as a cost containment tool for reducing inventories and controlling lost charges in the various hospital departments.

The recruitment and retention of personnel is a commonly cited problem among small rural institutions. Saginaw General was able, in several instances, to provide substitute coverage upon the termination or extended absence of employees. One notable instance involved the Vice President of Saginaw General stepping into the void left by the termination of the administrator at Deckerville Hospital and taking over an important certificate-of-need request process to a successful completion. His assistance also was provided in a plant expansion program at another contracting institution.[17] Hills and Dales Community Hospital benefited by the temporary loan of a registered nurse to serve as Director of Nursing during a vacancy in that position.[18]

Despite a failure to implement the inhouse computer capacity and technical assistance program as intended, both the Harbor Beach and Deckerville Hospitals participate in an off-line computer linkage for payroll services through Saginaw General.[19]

The benefits of high volume, negotiated price, and group purchasing were originally realized through a process that featured Saginaw General as the central contracting purchaser and on-site vendor delivering to the participating hospitals. This system was replaced when the participating hospital purchasing agents reached a decision to enter jointly the Hospital Purchasing Service, a statewide group purchasing service for hospitals.[20]

Educational activities cross both the administrative and clinical areas. The Saginaw General Director of In-Service Education, in conjunction with her counterparts in the contracting hospitals, coordinates the in-service activities which involve sharing program designs and educational resources among the institutions. Administrators meet twice monthly in programs consisting of literature review and study, and problem solving activities. Educational activities for department heads are provided through periodic meetings and seminars usually led by the appropriate department head at Saginaw General. Trustee education seminars on such topics as the trustee's responsibility for the quality of care and proper role in the institutional planning process were held with personnel of Saginaw General, public agencies, and private consulting firms serving as faculty.[21] Members of the medical staffs of the contracting hospitals attend seminars sponsored by the Saginaw General medical staff.[22]

Certainly one of the more serious problems faced by small rural hospitals relates to their inability to provide certain types of clinical services. Several Operation Outreach hospitals faced such a problem with their anesthesia coverage. The problem was addressed through joint contracting for a certified registered nurse anesthetist by two hospitals. Hired and carried on the payroll of one hospital for use in both hospitals, the nurse anesthetist's contract also specified the prerogative of brokering his services to other hospitals as time permitted and need dictated.[23] A cardiac monitoring program shared between Saginaw General and the Deckerville Community Hospital is another example of such service improving capabilities.[24]

As indicated by most of the activities cited above, the processes developed were related more to "shared services" than to "management contracts." This development seems to have occurred in part by original design—it was proposed to share the expertise found in contracting hospitals in programwide activities—and in part as an adjustment to the fact that Saginaw General had been unable to attract new contracting hospitals. Saginaw General recognized this difficulty, reasoning that:

> As currently structured, the risk is too great and the costs—real or perceived—too high to encourage an incumbent administrator to become an employee of Saginaw General in order for his hospital to become a participant in Operation Outreach. [Consequently] we will adjust our entry requirements to encourage participation of a hospital which retains full control of the administrator.[25]

This adjustment in program structure and strategy is further apparent in a promotional description of the Operation Outreach program:

> It [Operation Outreach] is a *process* (not a product) . . . it is a *sharing* of services, methods, and resources of the participating hospitals (the majority of which are provided through Saginaw General Hospital) and not the *"selling"* of services by one hospital to another. [emphasis in original][26]

The program thus took on many of the characteristics of a shared service consortium (not unlike Virginia Mason or Henry Ford), while maintaining an orientation to the future development of more management contracts. It was Saginaw General's view that management contracts will develop in time from this less pervasive level of cooperation as familiarity and trust are nurtured and as more benefits are realized by the participants.[27]

One consequence of this adjustment was a shift in the locus of programmatic initiatives and, to a certain extent, overall direction of the Operation Outreach program. A Joint Advisory Board, made up of two board members from each of the affiliated hospitals and Saginaw General, was established to serve in an advisory capacity to the Director of Operation Outreach. It was felt that this vehicle would serve to promote greater reliance on input from participants in the identification of short-range goals. Final approval of goals and processes, however, remained with the Saginaw General board.[28]

Impact and Outcome

The experience thus far of the Operation Outreach program can best be described as mixed: successful application of certain programs and plans were realized along with a number of setbacks and readjustments in the direction and structure of the operation.

Midway through the grant period there was a recognition that the level of service activity provided from Saginaw General—in particular the level of one-time specific-problem consulting by Saginaw General staff as revealed by major amounts of budget surpluses for these services—was below desired levels. The Huron Memorial Hospital had expressed particular dissatisfaction in this regard. Saginaw General attempted to solve this problem by developing a hospital performance indicator and data collection effort, reasoning that the diagnosis of problem areas would provide better direction and impetus in the development and application of services.[30]

The disappointment registered at the Huron Memorial Hospital eventually resulted in that hospital's board withdrawing from the management contract program. One observer attributed this occurrence and other problems to deficient initial planning, lack of precontract assessment of problems, and a failure to clearly and effectively present the project to participating boards, the result of which was a lack of understanding as to commitments and scope of services.[31] Given this experience and the widely acknowledged sensitivities and concerns that accompany management contract agreements, careful attention to board education and involvement was noted as a necessary ingredient to a successful program. Initiation of a Joint Advisory Board is evidence of Saginaw General's recognition of this and is seen as a positive step in this direction.

Disappointment was also noted in the participation of physicians in program services and activities.[32] The greatest potential for their participation, as seen in several other management contract programs, may well lie in the area of continuing medical education. The Chief of Staff at Hills and Dales Community Hospital expressed these same sentiments in evaluating the potential of the Operation Outreach program.[33]

A number of positive results were experienced as well. A first year progress report contained the following summary statement:

> It has been repeatedly stated from individuals in the affiliate hospitals that perhaps the greatest identifiable impact which the program has had . . . is a change in attitude [in the hospitals]. The knowledge that information and assistance is readily available, that resources are available to the board, the administrator, and the department heads . . . has permitted the performance of activities to be conducted with a greater degree of assurance.[34]

The experience at Hills and Dales Community Hospital was a satisfying one for all concerned. The severe financial problems noted earlier were remedied within a year's time.[35] A board member reported that ". . . the hospital would probably have had a hard time surviving had it not been for the interest of Saginaw General to become associated with it."[36] The new administrator at Hills and Dales, in support of a widely cited benefit of the management contract model, the ability to attract management talent, acknowledged that had it not been for the contract relationship he would not have been interested in the position.

The Deckerville Community Hospital board also reported enthusiastically on the program, feeling that the life and vitality of their hospital had been assured by the relationship.[37]

Increased ability to cope with the variety of external agencies with which the hospital must relate has been another commonly cited advantage of multi-unit arrangements. In this regard, it is reported that the budgeting systems subcontracted to the Wayne State University group had performed effectively to enable the participating hospitals to meet the prospective reimbursement ceilings established by Michigan Blue Cross.[38] Further support of this assertion is provided by the action of the East Central Michigan Health Systems Agency which used the Operation Outreach Program as a model sharing arrangement, citing it as part of the area's 1978 Health Systems Plan.[39]

As noted, by early 1979, Operation Outreach had not attracted new members, but rather continued to operate with only the management contract arrangements discussed at the outset. However, the boards of the existing affiliates each voted unanimously to approve the budget for the upcoming fiscal year. This action would indicate at least the general satisfaction of the affiliates with the Operation Outreach program, particularly since this is the first year that Kellogg grant support will no longer be available. Fees charged from services will support over 80 percent of the budget with Saginaw General contributing the remainder.[40]

Reversing a previous strategy, it was decided to discontinue efforts to encourage the participation of nursing homes in the program. Discussions with nursing home administrators revealed that an association of county nursing home administrators in Michigan already offered needed support. The hospital orientation of existing Operation Outreach services and the costs involved also were seen as barriers to nursing home participation.[41]

The short-term agenda calls for discussions to begin with three hospitals in central Michigan, the purpose of which is to explore the desirability of affiliation with Operation Outreach. An alternative proposal, should this not come to pass, has Operation Outreach assisting these hospitals in seeking, as a group, a tertiary hospital in the Lansing area with which they might affiliate in a program distinct from Operation Outreach.[42] Thus, Operation Outreach would serve as a catalyst to encourage other interorganizational affiliations. In addition, increased marketing activities are anticipated in order to expand the number of participating institutions.

REFERENCES

1. "Operation Outreach: A Proposal to Provide Contract Management and Support Services to Michigan Thumb Area Hospitals." Submitted by the Saginaw General Hospital to the W. K. Kellogg Foundation, 1976.
2. Ibid.
3. Ibid.
4. Klicka, Karl S., M.D. "Field Notes: Saginaw General Hospital." April 18, 1977, consulting report to the W. K. Kellogg Foundation.
5. "Report to the W. K. Kellogg Foundation for the Second Year of a Three Year Grant," from the Saginaw General Hospital, July 5, 1978.
6. Ibid.
7. Ibid.
8. Ibid.
9. Georgeson, Robert. Saginaw General Hospital. "Response to W. K. Kellogg Foundation Letter of July 28, 1978," August 17, 1978.
10. Klicka, "Field Notes: Saginaw General Hospital . . ."
11. "Operation Outreach: A Proposal to Provide Contract Management . . ."
12. Ibid.
13. Ibid.
14. DeVries, Robert A. *Program Notes:* W. K. Kellogg Foundation, 1976.
15. "Operation Outreach: A Proposal to Provide Contract Management . . ."
16. "Report to the W. K. Kellogg Foundation," from Saginaw General Hospital.
17. "Report to the W. K. Kellogg Foundation for the Second Year . . ."
18. Ibid.
19. "Report to the W. K. Kellogg Foundation," from Saginaw General Hospital.
20. Ibid.
21. "Report to the W. K. Kellogg Foundation for the Second Year . . ."
22. "Operation Outreach: A Proposal to Provide Contract Management . . ."
23. "Report to the W. K. Kellogg Foundation for the Second Year . . ."
24. "Report to the W. K. Kellogg Foundation," from Saginaw General Hospital.
25. "Report to the W. K. Kellogg Foundation for the Second Year . . ."
26. Ibid.
27. Georgeson, "Response to W. K. Kellogg Foundation Letter . . ."
28. "Report to the W. K. Kellogg Foundation," from Saginaw General Hospital.
29. Klicka, "Field Notes: Saginaw General Hospital . . ."
30. "Report to the W. K. Kellogg Foundation for the Second Year . . ."
31. Klicka, "Field Notes: Saginaw General Hospital . . ."
32. "Report to the W. K. Kellogg Foundation for the Second Year . . ."
33. Klicka, "Field Notes: Saginaw General Hospital . . ."
34. "Report to the W. K. Kellogg Foundation," from Saginaw General Hospital.
35. "Operation Outreach: A Proposal to Provide Contract Management . . ."
36. Klicka, "Field Notes: Saginaw General Hospital . . ."
37. Ibid.

38. "Report to the W. K. Kellogg Foundation for the Second Year . . ."
39. Georgeson, R. "Response to W. K. Kellogg Foundation Letter . . ."
40. Georgeson, Robert W. Operation Outreach. Letter to John M. Lowe, III, W. K. Kellogg Foundation, February 21, 1979.
41. Ibid.
42. Ibid.

Virginia Mason Medical Center
Health Services Consortium

Background and Structure

The origin of the Health Services Consortium is illustrative of the response to severe institutional need that characterizes the development of many multi-unit arrangements. Willapa Harbor Hospital, a 39 bed rural hospital 120 miles from Seattle, had lost three of five staff physicians within a four month period. The root of the problem was that the community had too few medical and education resources to attract or retain physicians. The hospital turned to the Washington/Alaska Regional Medical Program (W/ARMP) for assistance in the problem. In 1970, the W/ARMP called upon Virginia Mason Hospital in Seattle, which agreed to assist. Shortly thereafter, Virginia Mason was able to recruit a physician and a MEDEX-trained physician's assistant to the Willapa Harbor staff.[1]

With modest start-up support from the W/ARMP, the relationship between Willapa Harbor Hospital and Virginia Mason continued as a pilot project to investigate the capability of such an arrangement between a sophisticated urban medical center and a rural hospital to meet the considerable needs of rural hospitals. In Washington State, physician shortages, lack of training opportunities for health professionals, and gaps in continuity of care were being reported with some frequency in the rural settings.[2] Furthermore, close to 50 percent of all the hospitals in Washington operated less than 50 beds.[3] Upon completion of the pilot project, W/ARMP concluded that the arrangement was successful in increasing access to quality health care for rural citizens, in improving the rationality of physician referral systems, and in representing the first step in the development of informally regionalized health services.[4]

Taking on the name of the Health Services Consortium, by 1973 the arrangement had expanded to include seven other hospitals. Impetus for the collaboration had originated with specific requests for assistance from these other hospitals to Virginia Mason. Excluding Virginia Mason, the average size of the Health Services Consortium hospitals was 49 beds, ranging in distance to Seattle from 76 to 160 miles. Virginia Mason itself was, at the time, a 300 bed general hospital, the central institution in the Virginia Mason Medical Center. The Medical Center included the Mason Clinic, a multispecialty fee-for-service group practice of approximately 80 physicians practicing in a facility adjoining the hospital, and the Virginia Mason Research Center, a clinical research group operating at an annual budget of approximately $1 million. Virginia Mason had an active medical staff of 110 physicians of which only 15 were general practitioners.[5]

In short, Health Services Consortium may best be described as a professional and administrative support urban-rural shared services consortium.[6] It is based upon the notion of a consortium as "a group of institutions of an area voluntarily joined together to achieve *specific* purposes."[7] Central to the concept is that it does not require that the participating institutions hold all major goals in common; rather, advantage is found in pursuing specific goals which the institutions do have in common. Aware that it is often difficult to expect voluntary arrangements to develop between a large urban hospital and small rural hospitals in a region, Health Services Consortium took special interest to understand and articulate areas of common interest, incentives for cooperation, and barriers to collaboration in an attempt to establish a sound foundation upon which to frame the structure and guide the evolution of the consortium.

Several incentives were identified. From the viewpoint of the large sophisticated urban hospital, the consortium was seen to offer an ability to attract patient referrals. Virginia Mason, as the composition of its medical staff indicates, is essentially a specialized tertiary care facility, performing complicated procedures (e.g., open heart surgery) which requires a critical mass of volume to assure quality and cost-effectiveness. Also attractive from Virginia Mason's viewpoint was an ability to spread overhead costs over a wider base, to strengthen and expand their educational base, and to develop experience with an increased capability to cope with changes in the health care delivery system. Virginia Mason also felt that the consortium offered an opportunity to broaden the horizons of its supervisory and management personnel and enrich their job experience.[8]

From the viewpoint of the small rural institution, incentives commonly cited in the literature of such arrangements were identified: access to multiple services and resources, an increased ability to attract health professionals, improved quality of care through easier referrals, and strengthening the institution's image in its community by fostering confidence that it can meet the medical care needs of that community.[9]

As well as incentives, certain barriers were noted. From the urban hospital's viewpoint, concerns were expressed in the following areas: possible depletion of medical center resources, "backlash" created by the disruption of traditional referral patterns among physicians, and potential lack of urban hospital physician support. From the rural hospital's viewpoint, there were fears over loss of institutional autonomy, physician fears of the loss of patients following referral, professional sensitivities between rural general practitioners and urban specialists, and fears that financial support of the arrangement would put too much strain on already limited fiscal resources.[10]

Overall, there was an awareness of a potential for significant benefit tempered by several concerns, primarily in the areas of overtaxation of resources, physician acceptance, and institutional autonomy. The development and choice of what is described as the consortium model is a logical outgrowth and manifestation of these concerns. The structure has been designed to emphasize integration, coordination, communication, cooperation, and interdependency among member organizations.[11] In this regard it should be noted that there were no contractual arrangements between the participating hospitals in the Health Services Consortium other than letters of agreement on certain principles. In the words of a participant, " . . . we don't need a formal legal contract, for the inherent merits of the program will keep us together."[12] The loose structure of the consortium was additionally seen as beneficial in allowing the flexibility necessary to adapt to future pressures and changes in the industry as a whole, and in the hospitals and communities served.[13] Thus, the participants in the development of Health Services Consortium saw considerable advantage in adopting the consortium model as the means to test what was, for each of them, uncharted waters.

It is instructive to review the consortium objectives and operating guidelines with an eye towards the concerns of autonomy and flexibility. The preamble to the *Organization and Operation Guidelines* adopted by the consortium serves as a formal statement of the purpose of the Health Services Consortium:

> ... to demonstrate the viability of voluntary shared service relationShips between urban and community hospitals which will improve patient care and expand resources and capabilities for the local community.[14]

Seven operational objectives were specified:[15]

1. Promote greater continuity of patient care as a result of improved communication between referring and supporting participants.
2. Develop standardized quality checks for the major aspects of patient care and the results of in-service training.
3. Promote advancement of operational organization and cost control in both urban and rural hospitals.
4. Promote higher levels of professional and para-professional competence and education among participants.
5. Develop a viable and self-sustaining program.
6. Promote the principles of the consortium organization.
7. Maintain awareness and documentation of other derived benefits of the program.

In support of these objectives, five operating guidelines were established:[16]

1. We recognize that each hospital has the responsibility of defining its own needs and programs. The initiative must come from the individual hospital. It is not the responsibility of Virginia Mason Hospital to do all of the planning.
2. The sharing of facilities and resources is not limited to the participating hospitals. We intend fully to act as a "broker" in order to bring in other resources that are available in the metropolitan area which might be of advantage to all participants.
3. We stress continually that local autonomy is important to the program. We do not intend to disrupt local autonomy.
4. We believe the trustees and physicians must be heavily involved as the program matures and that contacts with . . . health planning . . . and other similar agencies must be maintained and strengthened.
5. We believe that as much "shoulder to shoulder" work must be done as possible and that this type of work should be, wherever possible, done within the community setting . . . .

Health Services Consortium's organizational structure is also representative of the diffuse sharing of decision-making authority that characterizes the consortium model. Final authority over participation in and support of Health Services Consortium decisions and programs remains with the governing board of each institution. The central operating body of the consortium is the Steering Committee. Made up of the administrators of all participating hospitals, this body sets consortium policy and determines program implementation. The Steering Committee also serves as the liaison body to the communities and outside agencies. Staff assistance is provided by a full-time Executive Director who reports to the Steering Committee. Provision is made in the organizational structure for physician input via the Ad Hoc Physicians Advisory Committee.[17] Support staff specialists, a Financial Analyst and an Education Coordinator, serve under the Executive Director in the Health Services Consortium central office.

Throughout its formative stages, Health Services Consortium relied for its financial support on a combination of external grants and internally generated funds. As mentioned, early grant support was provided by the Regional Medical Program. In late 1972, Health Services Consortium initiated a drive to support further regionalization and broaden its array of services. When the RMP program was dismantled, Health Services Consortium approached the W. K. Kellogg Foundation, which then provided grant support amounting to almost $87,000 over a three year period. This comprised approximately 50 percent of the total operating budget for the three year period. The grant was structured to offer support on a declining basis over the three year period with a target of financial self-sufficiency by the end of the third year. Virginia Mason acted as the consortium's fiscal agent and grantee throughout this period.[18] The three year grant period began with a total of six participating institutions.

In the early years of the program, participating hospitals paid an annual per bed assessment plus a quarterly membership fee. However, consistent with the consortium notion of equality among members, basic revenue needs currently are met through annual membership dues, equally divided among participants, and based on an annually approved budget. Fees for consultation services are made up of salary, fringe benefits, out-of-pocket, and travel expense components. Consultation charges are negotiated in advance of the service rendered.[19] As the source of most consortium services, Virginia Mason is compensated by Health Services Consortium for time spent by their staff in arranging and conducting classes and other programs. Health Services Consortium in turn bills the community hospitals.[20]

Implementation and Process

Entry into the consortium is a relatively straight-forward process. Informal personal networks and the consortium's monthly *Newsletter*, distributed to consortium members, local planning agencies, and other groups, serve to inform potential members and spur initial contacts. Potential candidates will pursue their interests with discussions with consortium members and by attendance at Steering Committee meetings. Applications for membership in the consortium are reviewed and acted upon by the Steering Committee. The Steering Committee reviews and judges applications with an eye towards such criteria as:[21]

1. Whether the hospital needs services or would supply resources.
2. The ability of the hospital to meet membership dues.
3. Proximity of the hospital to other member hospitals.
4. Commitment to the philosophy and purposes of the consortium.
5. Support of and participation from the applicant hospital's board of trustees and medical staff.

Such a review process is illustrative of the general decision-making process of Health Services Consortium. Proposals for joint or individual activities originate at the local hospital level and/or consortium level. As indicated in the guidelines for operation, considerable emphasis is placed on the initiative of the local hospital in order that their needs, as they see them, be met. In support of this initial step in the decision-making process, a study group evaluating the consortium recommended that each hospital develop a two year plan for participation as a guide to future programming.[22] Discussion and consideration of proposals then follow at the Steering Committee level or, if the proposal pertains only to a single institution, between Virginia Mason and the individual institution. If the proposals are acceptable, planning follows at the Steering Committee and staff level.[23] Implementation takes place with the assistance of a designated liaison person at the local hospital level. For example, an accepted proposal for a "teaching-treating" clinic at a local hospital will be coordinated and managed by a liaison physician at the local institution who serves as the official contact for the project.[24]

Projects or programs can be categorized into two types, according to the process by which they are initiated and implemented. The first category includes those that follow the formal process outlined above and that affect several or all of the consortium members. The other category includes those projects initiated on an informal basis, most likely by a telephone call, that are more in the nature of institution-specific requests for consultation assistance from Virginia Mason.

In the first category are those programs which relate primarily to quality of care concerns. Important among these is a cooperative medical audit program. This program was initiated upon request of the local community hospital physicians who found they had neither the time nor the staff to develop and implement a meaningful program alone. Audit criteria were developed by Virginia Mason medical staff with the local hospitals. The medical records administrator at Virginia Mason works with local hospital medical records personnel in reviewing completed audits and discussing variations from the criteria which are then conveyed to the various medical staffs for discussion and follow-up, a process consistent with JCAH requirements.[25]

Numerous other programs were established on a similar basis. A WATS telephone system was established whereby member hospital physicians can call Virginia Mason at no charge to receive consultation with the appropriate specialist. A variety of continuing medical education courses were established for the benefit of the local general practice physicians with an effort made to hold them in more accessible rural locations. Advanced nurse training in the areas of stroke and coronary care also was initiated.[26]

Of special note are two programs which give evidence of efforts to involve participants from local communities. One was an 85 hour Emergency Medical Technician training program in the community of each member hospital. In 1975, 170 people became certified as Emergency Medical Technicians by the Washington State Department of Social and Health Services through this program. The other program was a series of health education forums held in the member hospital communities. The forums dealt with topics such an hypertension, diabetes, and arthritis. Virginia Mason medical and nursing staffs were involved as faculty as were member of the local medical staffs.[27]

The second category, those initiated and implemented on an institution-specific basis, involved projects focusing on technical and management problems and tasks. Projects in this category included assistance in the recruitment of nurses, laboratory, and x-ray personnel.[28] Mentioned earlier was an example of assistance in the recruitment of a physician and physician assistant. Other examples are the coordination of Medline searches, comparative analysis of laboratory tests, and the loan of x-ray calibrating equipment. Specific requests for assistance in hospital rate analysis, wage and salary analysis, and development of hospital business office procedures also were answered. A pharmacy consultation addressed drug inventory policies and procedures in an attempt to lower costs.[29] One project in the fiscal area involved a data processing agreement whereby one of the small member hospitals used the computer services of Virginia Mason for patient billing, accounts receivable, aging analysis, and monthly billing reviews.[30] Thus far, most of the assistance or consultation has been provided directly by Virginia Mason. However, efforts are under way to encourage activities between rural hospitals directly.

Other programs, dealing with a variety of issues, are also provided. These include employee leadership seminars, respiratory therapy training, infection control classes, Accredited Record Technician preceptorships, electrical safety qualification consultations, team nursing conferences, and medical resident preceptorships at the rural locations.

Impact and Outcome

One indicator of overall satisfaction and success has been Health Services Consortium's ability to increase and retain its membership. During the three year period of the Kellogg Foundation support, Health Services Consortium grew from 6 to 10 members. In addition, the level of program activity increased continuously through the period.[31] Programs have been initiated by different groups, have dealt with a broad array of problems, and have led to a variety of strategies for resolution.

Also important is the continued financial commitment to the consortium by its members. Throughout the grant period, the consortium progressively assumed more and more responsibility for supporting the budget with internally generated funds. The target of self-sufficiency by the end of the grant period was met by Steering Committee action to increase membership fees.[32] These actions suggest that the benefits were perceived to outweigh the costs by those trustees and administrators responsible for each institution's resources. During the period, mechanisms were developed for local hospital governing board education to assure that trustees become familiar enough with the system so as to utilize it effectively and to support its continuation.[34]

Health Services Consortium has also had an effect upon other organizations with interest in multi-institutional arrangments. Following a visit to Seattle to study the Health Services Consortium arrangement, St. Joseph's Hospital in Albuquerque, New Mexico developed a similar organization of eight hospitals in 1976. Health Services Consortium reports that St. Joseph's decision to develop that arrangement was a direct result of their visit.[34]

As indicated, there were apprehensions over the loss of institutional autonomy and control during the initial formative period. A survey evaluation funded by the Kellogg Foundation following the first year of its grant support addressed this question. Responses by trustees, administrators, physicians, and other management staff members were "unanimous" in expressing the judgement that there is no loss of autonomy or control over institutional destiny. In fact, many felt that their institutions were more secure and independent in that they now possessed access to resources which gave them increased capacity and capability to deal with the problems facing their institutions.[35]

The increased access to and availability of services and personnel, brought about by the formation of Health Services Consortium, has implications for the quality of care and for the capabilities of those providing patient care. Continuing medical education and other health professional training comprised a large portion of the consortium's activities and were well supported and attended.[36] The initiation and growth of the cooperative medical audit program is seen as a step favorably affecting the quality of care. The WATS telephone consultation system saw dramatic growth from 566 consultations in the second year of grant support to 1,446 in the third. An effective referral system works to assure that patients receive care at the proper level and type of setting along with assuring continuity of care. Such is part of the justification behind regionalized health care systems. While it is not entirely clear that referral patterns were affected significantly by Health Services Consortium in the western Washington State area, the Puget Sound Health Systems Agency reported that Health Services Consortium " . . . meets the *Regionalized System* specification in the *Hospital Development Guide for Central Puget Sound*, providing a model of regionalization for other hospitals."[38] Where referrals did take place, the consensus of those involved was that the timeliness and quality of referral documentation was significantly improved.[39] Nursing directors in institutions where advanced nurse training took place expressed the opinion that more complete patient charting and improved communications between nursing and medical staffs resulted.[40] It was on the basis of findings such as these that the initial survey concluded that patient care was the area where the impact of the consortium has been most worthwhile.[41]

One of the potential barriers to arrangements between urban and rural institutions was said to relate to the "sensitivities" of the rural physicians and the potential for lack of support by the urban physicians. Indications are that these fears have not materialized. On the contrary, rural physician "sensitivities" have been reduced as closer professional relationships developed between the two groups of physicians. The urban physcians, rather than criticizing the practices of their rural counterparts, have shown an attitude of willingness to assist, as evidenced by their involvement in the continuing medical education programs, which have been designed to maximize utility at the local level.[42] Fear of the loss of patients during the referral process, an initial concern of the rural practitioners, has been overcome through experience with the process. Several factors are felt to have contributed to this development. For one, the institutions and office practices of the rural communities are sufficiently distant from the city so that patients are not apt to forsake their local community for care in the city. In addition, the levels of care practiced in the city and rural settings have been more complementary than substitutable, so that Virginia Mason finds it in their interest to rely on the community hospitals and physicians for primary care.[43] Another indication of support is evidenced by examples of program requests initiated by physicians.

In the area of cost control, several cases of savings have been identified. A drug inventory reduction in one hospital was estimated to have saved $2,000-4,000 at a cost of $900 for the consultation that brought about the reduction.[44] In another institution, $400 per year was the estimated savings resulting from a change in an x-ray filing system.[45] For the most part, however, there has not been evidence of widespread cost savings. Still, Health Services Consortium feels that cost control ideas previously considered by the individual institutions on their own but which were never implemented may be more likely to come about given the expertise made available through the consortium.[46]

Recent developments at Health Services Consortium indicate that the organization may be evolving toward more pervasive types of arrangements. In 1977, the administrator at one of the community hospitals became ill, requiring an extended absence from his hospital. Through Health Services Consortium, Virginia Mason made one of their administrative staff available to that hospital for the interim. When the original administrator was unable to return, a decision was made by the governing board of the hospital to hire the interim administrator who would be employed by Virginia Mason and serve the community hospital through a contract between Virginia Mason and the hospital. As of mid-1978, three Health Services Consortium hospitals were involved in such arrangements.[47] Referred to as "administrative service agreements," Health Services Consortium distinguishes such agreements as having a lesser degree of " . . . direct internal involvement and control . . . "[48] when compared to management contracts. The key point, however, is that this evolution suggests the satisfaction and confidence among participants which has arisen from prior arrangements.

REFERENCES

1. "Seattle's Consortium for Education." *Modern Healthcare*, April 1974, p. 120
2. W. K. Kellogg Foundation. "Description of Health Services Consortium."
3. Ibid.
4. DeVries, Robert A. "Regionalization of Health Services in Western Washington State: Virginia Mason Medical Center and Seven Rural Hospitals." *Program Notes:* W. K. Kellogg Foundation.
5. DeVries, Robert A. "Field Notes: Western Washington State Regional Health Services Project, Virginia Mason Medical Center, Seattle, June 21, 1973."
6. DeVries, "Regionalization of Health Services . . ."
7. Boyle, Robert L. and Lundberg, Keith R. "Description and Analysis of the Health Services Consortium in Washington State - Regional Shared Services." Presented to Rural Health Conference, Oregon Medical Association, March 2-3, 1979, Sun River, Oregon.
8. Ross, Austin. Virginia Mason Medical Center. Correspondence to Robert A. DeVries, W. K. Kellogg Foundation.
9. Ibid.
10. Ibid.
11. Boyle and Lundberg.
12. DeVries, "Field Notes: Western Washington State Regional Health Services Project . . ."
13. Jones, Richard F. "Health Services Consortium First Year Program Evaluation." (unpublished) March 1975.
14. "First Year Progress Report of the Health Services Consortium to the W. K. Kellogg Foundation, 1973-74."
15. Jones, "Health Services Consortium . . ."
16. Ross, Correspondence to Robert A. DeVries, W. K. Kellogg Foundation.
17. "First Year Progress Report . . ."
18. DeVries, "Regionalization of Health Services . . ." *Program Notes:* W. K. Kellogg Foundation.
19. Ibid.
20. "Seattle's Consortium for Education," p. 121.
21. "First Year Progress Report . . ."
22. Jones, "Health Services Consortium . . ."
23. "First Year Progress Report . . ."
24. DeVries, "Field Notes: Western Washington State Regional Health Services Project . . ."
25. "First Year Progress Report . . ."
26. Ibid.
27. "Second Year Progress Report of the Health Services Consortium to the W. K. Kellogg Foundation, 1974-75."
28. "First Year Progress Report . . ."
29. Ibid.
30. "Second Year Progress Report . . ."
31. "Third Year Progress Report of the Health Services Consortium to the W. K. Kellogg Foundation, 1975-76."

32. Ibid.
33. Jones, "Health Services Consortium . . ."
34. "Third Year Progress Report . . ."
35. Jones, "Health Services Consortium . . ."
36. "Third Year Progress Report . . ."
37. Ibid.
38. Ibid.
39. Jones, "Health Services Consortium . . ."
40. Ibid.
41. Ibid.
42. Ibid.
43. W. K. Kellogg Foundation, "Description of Health Services Consortium."
44. "Seattle's Consortium for Education," p. 120.
45. Jones, "Health Service Consortium . . ."
46. Ibid.
47. Ross, Austin. Letter to Robert A. DeVries.
48. Boyle and Lundberg.

Summary

These case descriptions have reviewed the development of 10 multi-institutional systems, which were supported by grant funding from the W. K. Kellogg Foundation. These systems have evolved using a variety of organizational models and structures. For purposes of the preceding discussions, emphasis was placed on institutional relationships involving shared services, management contracts, and leases, arrangements which formed the basis for Kellogg funding. It is noteworthy that in almost all of the cases the organizations which became involved with these systems were small, rural facilities, operating under severe financial, manpower, and service capability constraints. As indicated earlier, assessing the impact of these systems is made difficult by data problems and, in several instances, by the short period of time in which the systems have existed. However, a number of observations are in order.

In terms of economic benefits, it is clear that the interorganizational arrangements described have resulted in the restoration of the financial health of the institutions served. This has been accomplished largely through improved internal operating systems and procedures which were introduced by management and financial specialists available via the system-level organization. Results have included increased revenue from third party payers, better collections and accounts receivables management, greater revenue and expense controls, and new budgeting systems. In several instances, the strength of the systems has been of value in gain-ing access to previously unavailable capital. Some cost savings for the systems have been indicated, notably through joint purchasing activities and through increased operating efficiencies. For the most part, however, cost savings have not been substantial as the cost of increased service capabilities in the affiliated institutions serves to offset savings for the system, at least for the period covered by this review.

Manpower benefits have been reported in the administrative and the clinical areas. The availability of management expertise, in a variety of functional areas, has contributed to the viability of many of the affiliated institutions. Successful recruitment of administrative personnel, both at the system and the institutional level, has been demonstrated. Functional specialists have been attracted to these systems, and, for the most part, institutional administrators have been located and placed in managed or leased facilities. Retention of such administrators has been posed as a potential problem, especially in those systems lacking a range of different types and sizes of institutions, which would thus limit job mobility. Recruitment of physicians and other clinical manpower appears to have been enhanced by the introduction of the systems. Availability of resources through the system is a positive incentive in the manpower recruitment effort. In addition, the presence of an upgraded management capability has proved beneficial in attracting health manpower.

Access to specialized personnel and the presence of previously unavailable health manpower has implications for the quality of patient care. There are repeated indications that both structural and procedural improvements were made which were believed to enhance the quality of care. Any number of illustrations of the achievement of JCAH accreditation, previously denied or not even sought, were offered. Development of continuing education programs for a broad array of health professionals is seen as contributing to an increased capability to deliver services.

As to organizational benefits, it is obvious that the systems have grown and expanded as a result of new arrangements. New markets have been penetrated, service areas have been expanded for the delivery of services, and new opportunities to use clinical and management capacity have been made available. It is less clear, however, that new referral networks have evolved for those systems based in large, urban hospitals. For the managed or leased hospitals, and the communities they serve, substantial benefits have accrued. In a number of cases, the very survival of the institution has resulted. For the institutions and communities, there is evidence of increased access to and availability of services and manpower, and a broader range of services provided. However, the nature of the integrations, to a large extent, has been horizontal, thus the communities served are not as yet able to accrue the benefits of vertical integration as well. A number of the systems are moving or are planning to move toward such vertical integration, and such issues undoubtedly will become part of the long-range planning agenda as new roles for the systems and their affiliates evolve.

In securing these benefits, the systems described have employed somewhat differing strategies as well as structures. Recognizing the long-standing hospital tradition of local control and autonomy, many of these systems have taken a low-key approach to marketing. Indeed, one could argue that this recognition is partly responsible for the evolution of the types of structures, e.g., management contracts, which retain ownership prerogatives and attempt to maximize local control while achieving the advantages of large-scale systems. In the same context, acknowledging the potential of local boards of trustees, physicians, and administrators to serve as barriers to the growth of systems has led, in many instances, to substantial educational efforts aimed at these groups. To a large extent, the reaction of and acceptance by trustees and physicians has been favorable. Several of the systems have found that, particularly in the start-up phases, early successes are invaluable both in overcoming potential resistance and in winning new constituencies within the organization and in the communities. These efforts also have been beneficial in attracting additional affiliates. In the same vein, the systems appear to be becoming increasingly selective in terms of potential affiliated organizations. Emphasis on pre-agreement evaluations, designed to test the feasibility of an interorganizational arrangement, identify areas which will require attention, and make the weaknesses known to both parties, is receiving greater attention. This step should serve to bring into accord the mutual expectations of the organizations involved.

On balance, then, the systems described have demonstrated achievement of a number of economic, manpower, and organizational benefits. The manpower and organizational benefits have been the more substantial thus far, suggesting that increased service capability, particularly for the small, rural hospital, has been the predominant force. This expansion of service capability, coupled with the infusion of clinical and management talent, has tended to offset much of the potential immediate economic benefit. Leaders of these systems believe, however, that over time their efforts will indeed yield significant economic advantages as well, bringing the performance of their systems more completely aligned with their promise.

Part III

Selected Conference Papers

The Issues Facing Multihospital Systems

*Robert M. Sigmond**

Hospitals' Future Role

The issues facing multihospital systems in 1978 all reflect the key question facing each of the individual hospitals which make up the multihospital systems: How does that hospital move forward to play an appropriate role in a comprehensive health delivery system in its own community?

The future of every single hospital–whether or not it is a unit of a multihospital system–will depend on how it addresses this key question during the remainder of the 20th century. Those which are not able to do so will lose their identity.

If most hospitals are not able to establish identity as leading agencies in community health delivery systems, then hospitals as we have known them will become a thing of the past, as has already happened in England. Instead of vital community institutions, they will become little more than collections of technical resources in a broader organizational framework; important resources but with little power of innovation and self-determination in community service, and little for hospital management to do of any importance.

* Advisor on Hospital Affairs, Blue Cross/Blue Shield Associations. Based on an address delivered at the Sixth Annual Invitational Conference on Multihospital Systems, 1978.

Multihospital systems which are not able to provide leadership in the evolution of the hospital role in comprehensive community health delivery systems may achieve some short-term gains, but they too will not survive.

The nation is inevitably moving toward comprehensive community health delivery systems–tortuously, painfully, but inevitably. Multihospital systems can facilitate this process. They can smooth the way, lead the way, by formulating their missions in terms of community health delivery systems. The opportunity is great. But, if multihospital systems attempt to compete with evolving comprehensive community health delivery systems–to present a choice between highly structured hospital support systems and less structured community systems–they will create much turmoil, but will eventually inevitably lose out.

There are many forces in our society working against a dynamic role for the individual hospital as a community institution–as contrasted with simply a collection of technical resources whose costs must be contained. These include many HSAs, most national policymakers, most academicians, and most financing agencies. The existing imbalance of power within most hospitals at this time–more directly concerned with well-run technology than with well people–also supports the subservient technical resources outcome.

But there are important exceptions. In his Arthur C. Bachmeyer lecture before the American College of Hospital Administrators last year, Walter J. McNerney challenged community hospitals to assume a more dynamic role in community health service delivery. In his Parker B. Frances Foundation lecture at the recent AHA meetings in Atlanta, Harvard's Howard H. Hiatt challenged the hospital to serve as the leading change agent in the evolution of effective community health delivery systems. Most important of all, the House of Delegates of the American Hospital Association at those same meetings adopted a clear-cut policy statement concerning the role of the hospital "as the key organizational component . . . for the delivery of health services in the community."

The fact is that, as Churchill said about democracy, the hospital is the worst possible *institutional* framework for leadership in organizing community health service delivery systems–except for all the alternatives available in most communities. Think about that one. Is there a better alternative in your community that the Health Systems Agency can turn to for such leadership? How long will it take for the Health Systems Agency to develop the resources and mandate as the Health Systems Authority?

Hospital Leadership

In my opinion, the time has come for hospitals all over this land to begin to move energetically to provide effective leadership in their own communities in the evolution of community health delivery systems–which incidentally if properly done, will necessarily be cost effective, will put cost containment in an appropriate health delivery context, and will fulfill hospital commitments to the Voluntary Effort.

For a wide variety of reasons, the leadership for this movement will come largely from the multihospital systems. Most individual hospitals, by themselves, do not have sufficient systemswide experience or sufficiently strong internal systems and common leadership commitment to begin to attack the problem. Multihospital systems can take the lead, and can succeed, but only based on a clear understanding of individual hospital development, their hangups and their important assets and resources.

Viewed historically, the situation facing most hospitals in 1978 is very similar to that which faced hospitals 60 years ago in 1918. In 1918, hospitals had clearly emerged from being places of last resort for the poor and dying, to become doctors' workshops with a wide range of services which individual physicians could use in serving rich and poor alike. But in 1918, the hospital had not yet assumed *institutional* responsibility for the organization and management of these complex medical services. They were still organized as doctors' workshops. The very complexity of the services the hospitals were then providing required better training of medical specialists and more systematic standards and control mechanisms within hospitals, but these did not yet exist. The leadership was assumed–not by the American Hospital Association or American Medical Association–but by the American College of Surgeons, which established a hospital standardization and approval program focusing on the medical staff and medical records, but holding the hospital–as an institution–ultimately accountable, rather than the individual physician or department heads. You all know–or should know–the story of the beginnings of this effort. Very basic standards–that almost everyone could accept in principle–were adopted. But so few hospitals measured up that the ACS burned the earliest records. In 1918, when the first annual survey was made, only 89 hospitals in the entire country could meet the relatively simple qualifications for approval. From this early beginning, against great odds and on a purely voluntary basis, with the leadership of the ACS for over 35 years, the hospital emerged as the institutional professional service center which it is today. The job is now being carried on by the ACS successor agency, the JCAH, which incidentally itself is now feeling the strains of the new health delivery system pressures on hospitals–and not as yet showing signs of rising to the occasion.

In 1918, most hospitals were not able–on their own–to face up to the fact that their stated mission, their governance, their organizational structure, and their performance did not come close to measuring up to the standards that 20 years of changes in technology and science and society made imperative. National leadership from the ACS was required to effect these changes–which came about at each hospital slowly but surely over decades, often in the face of indifference or strong opposition of important medical leaders at many hospitals. Many of you know that the fundamental concepts of the JCAH program are not fully accepted even today by some members of many hospital medical staffs. But the typical hospital faces its institutional responsibilities for quality care largely because of the efforts of a prestigious voluntary external agency–the ACS–which dealt with each hospital's development with sensitivity and toughness, with standards and with respect.

Today, the primary issue is no longer the organization of the hospital for quality care, although that issue is not yet–and probably never will be–totally resolved. Today, the primary issue is the development of the hospital as the key organizational component in community health delivery systems. As with the quality issue after World War I, this issue has been talked about for years–even decades–as the social, technological, and economic forces have all pointed to a new definition of hospital mission, starting at the national level 30 years ago with the report of the Commission on Hospital Care.

Still, most hospital medical staffs and boards of trustees–not to mention the chief executive officer in many cases–do not yet understand or accept the concept of a broader role for hospitals, which necessarily raises new questions about the hospital's mission, governance, organization, program elements, community relationships, and system relationships–the whole works. Most hospitals today do not begin to measure up to the most basic standards of a leading community agency involved in health delivery systems.

If the AHA's new PIER program–the Program for Institutional Effectiveness Review–about which you will be hearing so much in the next few years–includes the most elementary standards of hospital organization for community delivery effectiveness, they too will probably burn the records of their initial surveys.

As we face this issue in 1978, there is little likelihood that leadership will come from the American College of Surgeons, nor is it likely to come from the American College of Hospital Administrators at this time in their leadership transition. I suggest that the leadership–by and large–will have to come from the multihospital systems, using the AHA's new Center for Multihospital Systems as their coordinating mechanism.

There is a variety of reasons why an individual hospital has an almost impossible task, facing up–all by itself–to the development of a modern role in community health service delivery, as contrasted with carrying out this transition within the framework of a multihospital system. Some of the difficulties involve the problems for the individual institution in mobilizing the critical mass of highly specialized organizational and planning resources which are required. Other–more important–difficulties involve problems in maintaining continuing commitment to the changing role at the individual institutional level–as a variety of forces play themselves out in the relationships among trustees, management, medical staff, and various community agencies and interests.

Theoretically, an individual institution could supplement its own resources by contracting with a first class consulting firm–like the Healthcare Organization and Management Group; that's an unsolicited plug–and with a variety of shared services organizations for the outside resources required to become a key organizational component in its community's evolving health delivery system–and do it without becoming involved with a multihospital system. But that would be very difficult. As with the ACS 60 years ago, the typical hospital will require an ongoing commitment from an authoritative, respected organization, with visibility and credibility, which can provide sensitively but firmly, the guidance required to adapt every aspect of the organization to the new national standards that are required. Unfortunately, the HSA does not have the resources to do the job, although it can help if it understands. Hospital associations and academic centers and Blue Cross/Blue Shield Plans can help too, if they see the issue clearly, but they cannot do the job for most hospitals.

The transition that is required in the decades ahead will be much easier for hospitals which can associate themselves with forward looking multihospital systems. The challenge facing multihospital systems, then, is how to demonstrate to most hospitals that the multihospital system is the safest vehicle for traveling the treacherous road to the future. This will require two things of multihospital systems: (1) demonstration that any hospital already in a multihospital system has a clear-cut advantage in stable community health delivery system development, and (2) an individualized flexible marketing strategy that is responsive to the only thing that all hospitals have in common, namely, their knowledge that each one is different.

The Mission of a Multihospital System

Before going further in attempting to set forth the key issue facing multihospital systems, it is important to make it clear that most multihospital systems–the topic of this conference–are quite different from comprehensive community health delivery systems, although they may become the same under certain circumstances. The mission of health delivery systems relates directly to the health of people, only indirectly to the vitality of hospitals. The mission of a multihospital system relates directly to the vitality of hospitals, only indirectly to the health of people.

For the foreseeable future–as I see it–in comparison with multihospital systems, most community health delivery systems will be much looser organizationally, much more comprehensive in terms of the definition of health services, and much more narrowly focused geographically. For the foreseeable future, in comparison with community health delivery systems, most multihospital systems will–as in the past–tend to reflect much more explicit managerial accountabilities, a narrower definition of direct health service responsibilities, and a broader geographic focus. There may be important exceptions, but the general pattern will be one of a multihospital system developing support services to each of its hospitals, so that each hospital can play the most constructive role in the evolving health delivery system in its own community. In many situations, there will be little or no health delivery relationships between hospitals in the same multihospital system–as with the typical geographically dispersed Catholic hospital order today. In other situations, there will be clinical and delivery service relationships among some or all of the hospitals in the multihospital system, but these should not be very different from the relationships with independent institutions and agencies in the hospitals' geographic areas. Ideally, all hospitals in multihospital systems should also be leaders in community health delivery systems in their communities. The issue facing multihospital systems is how to move in that direction.

Multihospital systems do not–and cannot be expected to–meet the total health service requirement of a geographically defined population. Health services extend far beyond the reach of most hospitals. Multihospital systems can only address health service objectives to the extent that their various hospital units link up with other community systems in effective ways. Multihospital systems can–and should–organize to accomplish this goal.

AHA Policy Statements

Before developing the argument further, let us be clear on the individual hospital's role in health delivery–at least as clear as the AHA's House of Delegates was in 1977 when it adopted its policy statement[1] on this subject:

> *The Hospital*-its governing board, medical staff, administration, and health professional-*is the key organizational component for the delivery of health services in the community*. As a consequence, hospitals should be involved in the coordination and implementation of changes in the health system. Effective steps should be taken now by hospitals to organize themselves voluntarily in order to improve their capability to deliver comprehensive health services to the community.
>
> These activities will require coordination with physician and other health care entities in the community and can serve as building blocks toward the development of an improved delivery system. Many hospitals have already taken the leadership in developing consortiums for a variety of functions, while others have formed multi-institutional systems as a more highly structured mechanism to enhance efficient and effective operation and to expand access to a wider range of health services. Cooperative efforts in this regard can better meet the health care needs of the community, avoid unnecessary duplication, develop appropriate alternatives to inpatient care, and strive for proper utilization of health resources.
>
> Hospitals should become more knowledgeable about all health-related activities in the community. Careful appraisal by each institution of the community it intends to serve is essential. The institution should be aware of program decisions of neighboring institutions and of other proposed new programs in the community pertaining to health care services, facilities, health education, and manpower development. It should recognize its interdependence with other health organizations and community groups with health interests, and encourage continual creative interaction.
>
> The goals of the institution should be related to its resources and to the health needs of the people to be served. Because there are limited resources upon which to call, hospitals should participate with other institutions to distribute effectively those limited resources and, where resources are inadequate, to develop programs for raising additional funds.
>
> Hospitals should consider some of the following examples of joint activities that can assist in improving the health delivery system. Open discussion is a basic ingredient for success in all of the following activities.

The AHA's statement lists a dozen specific examples.
Now, let us be clear on what a comprehensive community health

delivery system is–at least as clear as the AHA's House of Delegates was in its 1977 policy statement:

> Although no single way of organizing medical and health care services in a community can be universally applied, certain characteristics of a more accessible and effective delivery system can be identified as long-range goals for the community. These include the provision of good quality comprehensive services on a coordinated and effective basis in geographic areas across the country. Comprehensive health delivery systems are those entities that embody these elements and can serve as models in the community as constructive change in the system is planned and developed. Hospitals should take initiatives and participate in systems for improving health care delivery.
>
> Such systems should bring together physicians, other health personnel, management, and facilities into a cohesive structure with the capacity to make available comprehensive health care to the community, either directly through a hospital's facilities and services or by contract with other health providers.
>
> Each system should identify its service area and should plan its services and facilities to meet the health needs of all those residing in that area. Geographically defining a service area will provide an opportunity to address problems of access to the disadvantaged and to underserved areas through these systems.

Well, those are the AHA's official policy statements defining the individual hospital's role, and defining comprehensive community health delivery systems. Unfortunately, the AHA has not yet provided a clear definition of a multi*hospital* system as contrasted with the Perloff Committee's emphasis, for example, on multi-*institutional* systems. As soon as feasible, the Center for Multihospital Systems should come up with useful definitions, based on the pioneering work of Bob DeVries, Monty Brown, Bob Toomey, and others.

By now, I hope it is clear why I do not see multihospital systems as necessarily synonymous with community health delivery systems. In most communities, the full range and complexity of community health service relationships will not be able to be forced into a corporate mold as suggested by the Perloff Committee's Health Care Corporation. But community health systems will require the leadership of hospitals with the kind of discipline and corporate resources that multihospital systems can provide.

Some may be disappointed that I don't see the future of multihospital corporations in terms of simply perfecting businesslike support systems within the multihospital corporation, taking an essentially neutral role in terms of community health systems development–leaving that up to the

HSAs or some other agency. Well, I just don't think that the social and community responsibility of a multihospital system can be less than the community and social responsibility of a single hospital, as outlined by the AHA's House of Delegates. There has to be a multiplier effect–not a neuter effect; otherwise multihospital systems will not be able to justify support from society. Very few multihospital systems have begun to face this kind of issue as yet. The time is now. Let's talk about what is involved.

To keep things simple, let's limit the discussion to multihospital systems–most of them today–in which there is little or no systematic community service or clinical relationships among the hospitals *within* the multihospital system; the relationships within the multihospital system are essentially between the headquarters and each individual hospital. The community service system relationships of each hospital lie outside the multihospital system. Actually, if we start with this basic model, it is not hard to develop the implications of more complex models, which require partial or complete community service systematic relationships within the multihospital system, but that is another paper for another day.

Re-evaluation of the System

As I see it, the key issue facing the type of multihospital system which I have described involves re-evaluation of every aspect of the system–mission, governance, organization, and services.

Mission

With respect to mission, there are few multihospital corporations which will not require a thorough revision of the corporate mission statement, based on an intensive and extensive planning process. Only through such a process will most multihospital corporations achieve a corporate understanding and commitment to the role of each of its hospitals as the key organizational component for health service delivery in its own community. No real purpose will be served if the process of revising the mission statement doesn't result in greater corporate commitment to the concept than was reflected by the members of the AHA House of Delegates when they embraced the concept. I doubt that very many of the delegates thought much about the immediate implications for his own institution and his own job. That is what is really required.

Governance

We know so little about hospital governance–how it works, how it can be strengthened, what its potential is–either in individual hospitals or multihospital systems! My inclination in this keynote address is to say nothing at all, and urge you to give a great deal of attention to the discussion by Sister Elizabeth Mary Burns and Carl Halvorson and Carl Platou at the concurrent session on Governance-and to put your two cents in. I will only say this much. Governance structures of multihospital systems should be designed primarily to strengthen individual hospital governance and to stimulate continuous constructive and creative tension between the governance of the individual hospital and its community delivery system as well as between the governance of the individual hospital and the multihospital system. Among other things, this will require new definitions of appropriate balance between inside and outside directors on multihospital system governing boards.

Organization

With respect to organization, I notice that the emphasis in your concurrent session at the conference will be on corporate office management structure.

From what I have been able to learn from my friends in organizational development,[2] that is an appropriate emphasis so long as it is carried out within the framework of some overall management and organization design configuration that can cope with such core problems as: (1) clarification of the specific mission of the system in relation to its hospital units, (2) managerial competence to identify and predict external pressures on the system and on its hospital units, (3) realistic planning processes, involving all relevant interest groups, (4) development of an over-all strategic plan with time-targeted operational objectives at multiple levels within the system and the hospitals, (5) organizational designs to cope with multiple and changing tasks, (6) increased emphasis on managing consensual decision making in an environment in which decision-making authority will become more–rather than less–blurred, and (7) coping with interunit and interorganizational conflict as a force for innovation rather than tension.

In complex organizations like multihospital systems, during a period in which the nature of the environment will necessarily be turbulent and uncertain, organizational development must necessarily emphasize what the O.D. chaps call organic characteristics as contrasted with mechanistic characteristics. In terms of organizational processes, this means participative decision making; open management and confrontation of conflicts, as contrasted with either authoritarian avoidance or resolution of conflicts; open, minimal time lag, minimal distortion communications; increased capability to quantify and optimize performance; and realistic approaches to risk taking. Organization will focus on new relationships of hospitals with people as well as patients, epidemiological approaches, and new relationships among health service and human service agencies.

Central Services

With respect to central services, I predict that the dynamic tensions involving centralization-decentralization will never be resolved in multihospital systems, but can become a source of continuing upgrading of performance.

The key point is that the multihospital system's central services be designed to help each of the individual hospitals to play the most constructive role in the evolution of each hospital's community health delivery system. The multihospital system's system must serve the hospitals; the hospitals should serve a community, not a multihospital system.

From this point of view, it is most desirable that as many central services as possible be separately priced and contracted, not only to hospitals within the multihospital systems but also to other hospitals and institutions not formally within the system. Central office services should include those which are most difficult for individual hospitals to provide for themselves or obtain effectively from organizations outside the multihospital corporation: policy development and planning processes, monitoring and evaluation; external relationships beyond the immediate community, especially with respect to government agencies, foundations, national recruitment, capital funds and technology, and staff development. Central systems involving accounting, data processing, engineering, purchasing, and the like can also be important, but not when they interfere with the ability of each hospital to work effectively with other community-based resources. Uniform reporting and budgeting procedures are, of course, essential. Beyond that, however, the value of conformity with uniform refined management processes throughout the system must be weighed in terms of the value of each hospital's ability to relate flexibly to its own constituency.

Role of the Medical Staff

You may notice that–in this general review–I have had little to say about the medical staff role and relationships within multihospital systems. Clearly the multihospital system must stand for significant involvement of the medical staff in policy development and management of the individual hospitals and of their increasing role in the hospitals' community health delivery systems. Beyond that, however, any specific role and relationship of hospital medical staffs of individual hospitals in a multihospital system without clinical service interrelationships is not at all clear to me. Here again, I look forward to the concurrent session–to what Jerry Hahn, Jack Skarupa and all of you have to say. It is a key issue.

*   *   *

I hope that these keynote remarks have achieved–to some extent–the following purposes: (1) to help to provide some historical perspective for your discussions of the next three days, (2) to challenge you to view your role in the broadest context possible within the framework of existing AHA policy, (3) to place the emphasis where I think it belongs–on the role of the multihospital system in helping the individual hospital to play a key role in community health delivery systems, (4) to see some logical pattern in the topics assigned for the discussion sessions to follow, and (5) to demonstrate clearly that each of us, especially me, has a lot to learn from the mutual exchanges of the next few days.

I cannot close without a personal note of appreciation to Gail Warden for his foresight in creating a Center for Multihospital Systems and for attracting Bob Toomey as its first consulting director. As I see it, this was an overdue step, in view of the growth of multihospital systems and their potential role in fulfillment of AHA policies.

Multihospital systems must grow and develop–because as Bob DeVries said–there is strength in numbers. Beyond that, they will grow and develop as necessary elements in this nation's structural foundations for comprehensive health service delivery. In so doing, multihospital systems will simultaneously relieve our metro, state, and national hospital associations of a large part of their crushing burdens, and enhance the likelihood that broad hospital association policy positions will be implemented in realistic ways. It is extremely difficult to imagine how very many hospitals in this country can meet the challenges reflected in current AHA policy–not to mention the challenges of a variety of other external forces–without multihospital system support.

REFERENCES

1. American Hospital Association. "The Provision of Health Services Under Universal Health Insurance." Statement approved by the AHA House of Delegates, August 30, 1977.
2. Tichy, N. and Beckhard, R. "Applied Behavioral Science for Health Administrators." MIT Sloan School of Management, Working Paper No. 879, 1976.

Generic Problems in the Development and Operation of Multihospital Systems

Edward J. Connors*

From 1974 to 1976, I have had the opportunity, as part of the Sisters of Mercy of Detroit, to study approximately 13 other systems with regard to purpose, organization, governance, management, and finance. Subsequently, I have had the experience of helping to design the Sisters of Mercy Health Corporation and, since 1976, to attempt to provide leadership for that organization–an organization that has been described as the largest voluntary, not-for-profit hospital system in the U.S. (exclusive of the Kaiser system).

With the insights gained from these experiences and my tenure as Chairperson of the Advisory Panel for the Center for Multihospital Systems, I have identified a few problem areas which I believe to be generic, fundamental, and highly relevant to all of us at this stage of the evolution of multihospital systems. These primary areas of concern are: (1) problems of achieving clarity of purpose and goals; (2) problems of developing leadership among multihospital systems with conceptual skills sufficient to develop the systems into positive, constructive change agents in the provision of health services; and (3) problems of achieving and maintaining governance and management structures that are adaptable, effective, and creditable to the people served.

* President, Sisters of Mercy Health Corporation. Based on an address delivered at the Sixth Annual Invitational Conference on Multihospital Systems, 1978.

Without attempting to make a case for systems, to cite successes, or to enumerate potentials, I shall examine these problems from a set of assumptions that includes:

- We are at the beginning of a long-term trend toward multihospital systems and arrangements.
- Multihospital systems have in the past and will, to a greater degree in the future, outperform the single freestanding organization.
- There will be much variation among and between systems. Pluralism will continue to characterize the ownership, financing, and operating approaches of multi-institutional arrangements.
- In the longer term, consortia, loose-sharing arrangements and mergers without teeth will give way to organizations with ownership obligations or tighter management arrangements, capable of committing an entire system to a course of action and direction of change.
- Competition will develop among and between systems, while at the same time there will be significant cooperation and joint effort.

Each of the problem areas evolving from this set of assumptions comprises a complex network of related issues and questions which will need to be carefully addressed in the near future. The initial task, however, is to delineate broad areas of concern and to pinpoint those questions that are crucial to the further development of hospital systems.

Problems of Achieving Clarity of Purpose and Goals

Multihospital organizations should be models of corporate planning. This requires that the central purpose or mission of the organization be explicitly stated, openly and widely promulgated, and determinant of goals, role options, and alternative objectives. However, many multihospital organizations seem to have evolved or emerged without the fundamental building block of clarity of purposes. A rush toward expansion, uncritical adoption of marketing techniques without a clear product to be marketed, and the desire by many to achieve a competitive edge seem to be all-too-common symptoms.

Developing a purpose through the process of discernment (or of conscious choice) requires that an organization examine the philosophies of those charged with the responsibility of establishing the mission or purpose of the organization. Philosophies, or basic beliefs, are likely to vary significantly among multihospital organizations. Some organizations reflect values stemming from religious ownership or preferences; others have a business efficiency and profit motivation; still others are products of a tradition of community based, not-for-profit leadership that has been a dominant feature of the American hospital scene; finally, others are expressions of governmental responsibility for the health of citizens governed. It seems important that these differences be recognized because, in fact, they become determinant of the central purpose and major characteristics of the organization. In many cases, current system leadership does not appear to have achieved the clarity so badly needed for significant growth and development at a time of rapid changes.

While the differences stemming from religious ownership, profit status, and community orientation are real and basic toward determination of purpose, there remains a significant number of issues to be faced concerning the organization, financing, and delivery of health care in this country. In light of the issues now extant and in harmony with the purpose developed for the organization, multihospital systems must respond, if they are to be models of corporate effort, by clearly enunciating goals, determining environmental factors affecting the organization, consciously developing objectives and alternate courses of action, and implementing a defined action plan. This process requires strategic planning on a corporate basis, utilizing in this context:

- *Goals*–the position, desired state, or level of performance to be achieved in fulfilling a purpose.
- *Objectives*–time honored and quantifiable measures of progress toward achievement.
- *Role*–the part to be played by the organization or individual hospital.
- *Strategy*–plan or method of achieving objectives.

It is through this basic process, all dependent on clarity of purpose, that multihospital systems have a chance to make a difference, to be on the cutting edge, to do something about the real and perceived problems plaguing the field of health services delivery. The challenge calls for the leadership of multihospital systems to rethink basic beliefs on such questions as:

- What is to be the role of government in financing, regulation, education of health professionals, and the provision of direct health services?
- What is believed to be the relationship between the scope and characteristics of health services provided on one hand and the health status of the people served on the other? How can multihospital systems have a positive impact on the health status of the people served? Can they have any impact? Is it their responsibility?

- What is to be the role of the health professional (physician, nurse, manager) in the functions of governance and management in a multihospital system?
- Of what value is the participation of local citizens in the governance decisions of a multihospital organization? How is that participation to be achieved–or avoided?
- What, in fact, is known or believed today about the reasons for the extreme variation in the utilization rates of the U.S. citizens (admission rates, days of care per 1,000 population per year, surgical rates)? In turn, what is perceived to be the relationship between the variation in use rates and the indicators of the quality of services provided? Do multihospital systems need to involve themselves in this variation except from a financial point of view?
- To what extent is there excess capacity (such as acute inpatient beds) and unneeded duplication of services and technologies? Are these perceptions of over bedding the current fad or are they of sufficient validity and impact to demand priority attention of multihospital systems?
- Is the nation committed to achieving comprehensiveness of services, with continuity, at acceptable levels of quality with predictable and supportable costs? If so, what are the strategies that can enable multiple hospital systems to achieve these laudable goals?

These questions are illustrative of the type of concerns and considerations that must permeate the thinking of multihospital systems if they are to take seriously the responsibility of corporate planning. Clarity of purpose and goals is fundamental to this process, but such clarity has not yet emerged with sufficient consistency among those responsible for organizing and directing multihospital operations.

Problems of Developing Leadership

Systems are emerging at a critical time in the development of our pluralistic health services. Many have been developed in recognition of the limitations of the single hospital, regardless of how extensively that individual hospital may have developed its own capacity to serve. As a result there are emerging vastly different organizational, financial, political, and management bases than have been available in the past. These new bases have greatly improved potential to respond to the signs of the time. The question facing multihospital systems is *whether* and *how* they wish to address the issues, the problems, and the weaknesses of our current array of activities loosely referred to as a health care delivery system.

At least two models of behavior are available to multihospital systems in responding to the opportunities of the times, and there are indicators that both models are represented and at work in any sampling of systems.

Efficiency Model

The first behavioral mode views itself as a model of efficiency. It applies the latest business techniques to current operations. Working hard on productivity indices and performance measures, it optimizes economies of scale in such endeavors as purchasing, cash management, and capital financing. This type avoids ventures with high financial risk such as ambulatory or long-term care and devotes political effort to maintaining the status quo with regard to reimbursement and regulation. By building a better mousetrap, this model hopes to penetrate the market and outcompete the neighboring hospitals. Government–or someone else–can care for the poor and near poor. The unmet needs of the served communities are not this model's concern, nor is containing costs as important as optimizing reimbursement. The greatest attention is given to being on the vanguard of technological diffusion because the latest equipment is likely to enhance the competitive edge.

Change Agent Model

The second model views itself as a vehicle to bring fundamental change in the delivery of health services. It works actively to achieve a coordinated, comprehensive plan of services for all the communities it serves. Thus it moves in the direction of developing ambulatory care centers with heavy emphasis on primary care, prevention, and health education. It converts excess bed capacity to ambulatory and long-term care services and to centers of health rather than to the treatment of illness. Collaboration with other providers achieves comprehensiveness and continuity of care at local levels, while concern with providing the appropriate number of beds and services rather than maintaining the current number ensures cost effective care. Acknowledging that there are problems of costs, quality, and access, this model designs specific goals and programs to deal with these problems. It makes sure that current and future utilization rates can stand the test of professional scrutiny and that variations are defensible. It actively works to eliminate the injustices that can be found in all of our communities, and it attempts to inculcate compassion and caring into the fiber and fabric of the organization. In short, it tries to be a value oriented enterprise even though these values may be working against the grain of some of our historical patterns.

Emerging hospital systems can and should make a conscious decision between these two oversimplified models of behavior–the Efficiency

Model and the Change Agent Model. These models are not discrete nor mutually exclusive; constructive change cannot be achieved without financial capability, for example. They are, however, dependent upon the leadership of the emerging multihospital systems. First and foremost, this leadership will require conceptual skills–the ability to see an enterprise or activity in its totality, to relate component parts to one another, and to understand the probable consequences of alternate courses of action. The generic problem is whether or not multihospital systems will emerge as constructive change agents. Will the leadership–those engaged in governance, the medical leadership, and those with management responsibilities–be able to convert their conceptual grasp of what their organizations are all about to the tangible impact so needed in our system. There are few if any other elements in the field of health with the opportunity and the potential capability to have such an impact.

Problems of Achieving and Maintaining Effective Governance and Management Structures

Governance has been a long neglected function of hospital administration. The voluntary not-for-profit single hospital model of governance was best developed by the time the mid 60s arrived—the time that signaled the development of multihospital systems on one hand and the widespread rejection of all institutions by the public, particularly the young, on the other. What sufficed for governance prior to the mid 60s is proving inadequate for the multihospital system, particularly the horizontally integrated system.

The response of multihospital systems to this governance question varies considerably. Some appear to have rejected local citizen participation in the policy issues of the organization in favor of what they deem to be greater corporate-wide authority and responsiveness. Relying on the abilities of the professional health executive and physician for important governance decisions, they seem to feel that government regulatory agencies can appropriately hear the voice of the citizen. Others are trying to build governance structures that will balance local initiative and responsibility with corporate responsibility and opportunity. They feel that strong citizen participation at the local level is a strength to be nurtured and integrated into the fabric of the organization. Governmentally operated systems are often plagued with no discrete governance mechanism, and some religiously oriented systems seem to be struggling with the advisory system and the relationship of church to governance.

All systems face difficult generic governance questions. They must, first of all, clearly define governance responsibilities and distinguish them from management responsibilities. They need to determine if the strengthened governance of multihospital systems will make them more credible to citizens served, to their owners or sponsors, to government, and to external agencies. They must ask whether trusteeship should remain a voluntary, unpaid function in view of the time required to become knowledgeable about the myriad of complex health care issues. They must also assess the role of the professional manager and the physician in trusteeship. Most importantly, they must determine which governance structure will be the most flexible and adaptable to the future growth and change that is inevitable for most systems, and which governance approach is most likely to achieve the change agent model previously described.

The successful implementation of the change agent model depends, to a large extent, on whether or not the managers of multihospital systems can understand and create the kind of environment where persons can and will perform to the optimum of their capability. Although management education has not always been wholly effective, much has been learned and developed about management practices in recent years. There has emerged a body of knowledge, a set of beliefs, and some hard evidence that management style does make a difference in effectiveness, productivity, and morale; that there are distinguishing characteristics of effective managers; that leaders of organizations can now make conscious choices on matters of management styles, processes, and policies; and that diagnostic and therapeutic tools exist that have advanced far beyond the fad or gimmick stage. The basic question is whether the leadership of multihospital systems will take advantage of the findings of the behavioral scientists in guiding and shaping these challenging new organizations.

Conclusion

The issue facing multihospital systems is not their ability to grow and expand. According to recent estimates, one-third of all hospitals and at least 40 percent of all community hospital beds are part of multihospital systems. In a nine year span, from 1968 to 1977, the number of hospitals grouped into systems and reported by the American Hospital Association grew from 200 to 2,300. Another survey shows existing nongovernmental systems growing 10 percent in 1978.

Rather, the issue is the ability of systems to recognize and respond creatively to the problems outlined here—problems of achieving clarity of purpose and goals, problems of developing leadership, and problems of building effective governance and management structures. Not until these problems have been squarely met can hospital systems achieve their full potential for becoming change agents in the delivery of health services.

Impact on and Opportunities for Multihospital Systems and Shared Service Organizations

*Donald C. Wegmiller**

Introduction

The purpose of this presentation is to discuss legislative and regulatory impact upon multihospital systems and, in addition, some description of how the systems may be of assistance in achieving the goals of health legislation and regulation.

The literature has adequately addressed the fact that Public Law 93-641, the National Health Planning and Resources Development Act of 1974, has as one of its overall goals the establishment of hospital systems. This is shown through an analysis of the 10 National Health Priorities established by Congress in Section 1502 where at least two of these priorities speak directly to the creation of multihospital systems and at least three speak indirectly toward the development of such systems. Previous speakers at this conference have clearly outlined those priorities.

Overview of This Presentation

I would like to cover with you the following topics on health legislation and regulation and their impact upon multihospital systems:

---

* President of Health Central, Inc. Based on an address delivered at the Invitational Conference on Multihospital Systems and Shared Services, 1978.

- The general climate of legislation and regulation in the health care field today, particularly from the viewpoint of the health care provider.
- Areas of difference or strength that multihospital systems do bring and can bring to the legislative and/or regulatory process.
- The application of existing and proposed laws and regulations to the development of multihospital systems, both positive and negative applications as seen from the hospital system's point of view.
- Some general issues of legislation and regulation in the areas of health finance, health planning, and quality of care.
- Finally, a summary of projections or suggestions for the future in the area of legislation and regulation and multihospital systems.

The General Climate of Legislation/Regulation in the Health Care Field Today

It is important to note that this description of the general legislative/regulative climate is from the viewpoint of a health care provider and particularly that of the multihospital systems in the health care field. Certainly different viewpoints are possible and are in existence.

It is also important to note that health care providers generally recognize and appreciate the need for some health care initiatives to come from legislation. These initiatives may deal with: problems of health underserving; specific areas of health care finance; health service projects which require testing or demonstration; or health care projects which require developmental funds beyond the scope of health care providers.

Health care providers also recognize and appreciate the need for *some* regulation to guide and implement the desired legislative health initiatives. Providers recognize that legislation cannot be implemented in an orderly, uniform manner without guidelines or planning efforts.

However, within this broad recognition and appreciation, health care providers feel that there are some problem areas with the general climate of that legislation and regulation today. Some of these problem areas include:

Symptom Type Legislation

Health legislation is many times directed at "symptoms" with little impact on "causes" and additionally is felt to be applied to hospitals with little regard for the other elements of society which are impacting upon hospitals. An example of this symptom type legislation is the current revenue containment legislation.

Although labeled cost containment legislation for political reasons, the legislation is clearly directed at containing the amount of revenue which flows into the hospital sector of the health care field. Therefore, the revenue containment legislation attacks the symptom of increasing expenditures without addressing the cause of increasing hospital costs of operation. Further, the legislation does not speak to any controls or containment of costs which are imposed on hospital operation from other elements of society which impact upon hospitals. This is but one example of symptom type legislation.

Regulatory Contradiction

The contradictory thrusts of health regulation is another problem area. Some of the examples of the regulatory contradiction include:

- The difficulty in reconciling the mandate from HEW to reduce or eliminate duplication of services in a common service area with the emerging mandate from the Justice Department for hospitals to be competitive in a common service area.
- HEW, operating under congressional direction of P.L. 93-641, currently urges the sharing of services between hospitals while Medicare reimbursement does not pay for the use of capital to develop these services. At the same time the IRS tax code taxes these sharing activities in many instances as unrelated business income or, in other instances, specifically forbids certain of the sharing services.

Antitrust Laws

There is considerable uncertainty in the health care field as to the application of antitrust laws to hospital operations, particularly those of multihospital systems. This uncertainty creates inertia and anxiety which, in turn, restricts development or retards development of needed changes in the health care delivery system.

Confusion About Regulations

The multiplicity, duplication, and conflict of regulation and the monitoring of those regulations by numerous agencies causes great confusion.

Volume of Regulations

The volume of federal regulations for all industries has increased tremendously in recent years. Table 1, depicts the mushrooming of federal regulations over the past 25 years. The overall increase in regulations has been paralleled by the increase in regulations affecting hospitals. Many federal, state, local, and voluntary agencies are engaged in regulation with which hospitals must be concerned. Table 2 is a matrix illustrating the types of regulatory activities affecting hospitals.

TABLE 1

Increases in Regulations Published in the Federal Register, 1950 - 1975

Year	Number of Regulations
1950	9,562
1960	14,479
1965	17,206
1970	20,036
1975	60,221

Lists of Regulations

Several state hospital associations have attempted to develop comprehensive lists of all regulations affecting hospitals. The Hospital Association of New York State (HANYS) reported in 1976 that 40 federal agencies, 96 state agencies, 18 city and county agencies, and 10 voluntary and quasi-public agencies—a total of 164 agencies—regulated some facet of hospital operations in New York. Many of these agencies performed their regulatory functions over a large number of areas. City and county health departments were reported as regulating 64 separate areas; the Bureau of Hospital Nursing Services of the state health department regulated 51; the Bureau of Nutrition of the same department, 48; the Office of Professional Standards Review, 48; and the Bureau of Hospital Certification, 45. These agencies constituted only a fraction of the total, and the wide scope of their authority was atypical.

In New York, 109 areas are regulated by more than one agency. Of the 109 areas, 82 are monitored by at least 10 different agencies. Reports and inspections on patients' rights are monitored by 33 agencies, 15 of which are state. Admitting procedures are reviewed by 25 agencies; 14 of which are state.

State Regulations

Not all states regulate their hospitals as extensively or intensively as New York, which is generally acknowledged as one of the states with the most wide-ranging and detailed set of regulatory controls. However, substantial burdens, including costs, may be imposed by efforts to comply even in the less heavily regulated states. Hospitals in Minnesota are required

TABLE 2
Regulation Grid

Regulatory Agency and Source of Authority Versus Elements Regulated

Agency or Program	Capital Construction	Costs-Charges Income	Institutional Personnel Standards	Professional Performance System of Review	Employee Conditions	Training	Patients' Rights	Accounting and Medical Records
Medicare	F	F	F	F	F	F	F	F
Medicaid (federal or state)	FS	FS	FS	FS	FS	FS	FS	FS
Public Health Service	F		F	F		F		
JCAH	P		P	P				P
Blue Cross Private Insurance	FSP	FSP	FSP	FSP				FSP
State insurance commissioner	S	S		S				
State Department of Health State licensing agency	FS		FS			FS		FS
Fire marshals	FS		FS					
NFPA	P		P					
Equal opportunity Department of Justice						F		
Courts						FS		
NLRB — Department of Labor State departments of labor					F			
State rate review		S						
Internal Revenue Service		F						F
Planning agency	FS							
PSRO				FSP				
AMA			P			P		
American College of Pathology			P					
AICPA (accountants)								P

F — federal, S — state, P — private.

Source: American Hospital Association. "Hospital Regulation: Report of the Special Committee on the Regulatory Process, 1977."

to conform to 20 regulatory programs in the area of institutional quality, 3 in manpower licensure, 2 in accreditation of health education programs, 4 in evaluating professional performance, 1 in controlling capital expenditures, 2 in health insurance, 2 in tax regulations, 11 in cost or price regulations, and 16 in labor laws. This is a total of 61 regulatory areas administered by 35 agencies. At least two agencies share regulatory responsibility for 16 of these areas.

Judgment of Inspectors

Regulation and inspection for compliance require the exercise of judgment by individual inspectors, and judgment can vary from one inspector to another. In some cases, the regulatory codes themselves are in such conflict that the same inspector applying two such codes produces radically different findings. In 1974, the Social Security Administration conducted a series of hospital inspections that were intended to "validate" earlier inspections of the same hospitals conducted by the Joint Commission on Accreditation of Hospitals. Recommendations and approvals made in the JCAH inspection were frequently negated by the SSA inspection. A study of the validation surveys of 97 of the hospitals indicated that the SSA teams made 4,300 recommendations, whereas the JCAH made 2,993 and only 7 percent of the recommendations were similar.[1] The differences were attributed to variation in size and composition of the inspection teams. The disparate findings were also attributed to reliance on different sets of standards, such as the use of different editions of the Life Safety Code of the National Fire Protection Association.

Areas of Difference or Strength Multihospital Systems Do Bring and Can Bring to the Legislative and/or Regulatory Process

Recognizing that the development of multihospital systems is a relatively recent phenomenon and the recognition of such systems by government and other sectors is also very recent, perhaps it is helpful to present some of the differences or strengths that these systems currently bring to the legislative process or can bring to the regulatory process. Some of these differences or strengths include:

- Systems are able to attract, retain, and afford increased staff specialists and expertise to understand and deal with the complicated regulatory process. This provides a better understanding of the regulations themselves, as well as a rationale behind the regulations. In addition, it provides for individuals in the delivery system with whom legislators and regulators can discuss goals of legislation and the purposes of the regulations. This additional understanding should result in a better interface between the goals of the legislation and its implementation by the health care field.

- The costs of compliance with regulation and legislation can be spread across a broader number of hospitals through the mechanism of multihospital systems. Uniform reporting techniques, and staff specialists in compliance in such areas as personnel, life safety regulations, building codes, and labor relations are examples of cost spreading areas available to multihospital systems.
- Since multihospital systems generally have a stronger economic and political structure, they have available and make more use of opportunities to participate directly in the legislative process. This is contrasted to the individual hospital's reliance on representation by trade associations and other groups. This direct participation should aid the legislative and regulatory process by a direct communication between the legislator/regulator and the health care provider. The sharing of ideas and opinions on the strengths and weaknesses of legislation and regulation should result in a better end product.
- Multihospital systems and their staffs can serve as resource groups for agencies to converse with on proposed legislation or regulation. The ability to converse directly with health care providers who represent numerous hospitals in a variety of settings (urban and rural, large and small hospitals, tertiary centers and community hospitals) can provide a variety of viewpoints upon which legislators and regulators can develop their health initiatives and regul tions. The sponsor of this conference, The Center for Multihospital Systems and Shared Service Organizations, is a new resource for just such conversations. Undoubtedly the Center will be in a position to coordinate such conversations.
- Systems can serve as somewhat controlled environments of more than one hospital in which various test programs might be conducted. These programs might be in such areas as health care reimbursement, quality controls, new forms of delivery patterns, medical care organization experiments, and the like.
- In that more than one hospital is controlled in the multihospital setting, opportunities for measuring the effectiveness of proposed regulation or legislation exists within these systems.

Usefulness of Differences or Strengths

As an example of how these differences or strengths of multihospital systems might be brought to bear, let's examine their usefulness in and potential effect on the currently proposed voluntary effort of cost containment mounted by the AHA, AMA, and Federation of American Hospitals. As you know, there is a 15 point program of voluntary cost containment efforts currently under way. There are at least 6 of those 15 points in which multihospital systems can more positively address the result than the single freestanding institution.

The first point in the voluntary effort is to create state level voluntary cost containment committees which will be the key element in these cost containment efforts. In setting up state level voluntary cost containment committees, the multihospital systems have the advantage of centralized management, and centralized governing boards which can plug into the voluntary effort through one staff covering a multiple of facilities. Where multiple facilities of a system reside in a specific medical service area, consolidated planning at the system level results in regional planning for the area contributing to reduction in duplicative services and in cost savings to the community. These efforts should be most important to the success of state level cost containment committees.

Another point in the voluntary effort is to significantly reduce new capital investment and to achieve a position of no net increase in total hospital beds for the next two years. By virtue of multiple facilities, capital investment in systems can be concentrated where services can be delivered in the most cost effective manner. Pooled capital has resulted in a lowering of debt financing requirements as well as more favorable interest rates resulting from pooling of assets. The results are a savings in interest expense passed on to the consumer in lower operating costs and charges. Many hospital systems also have consolidated capital budgets as well as pooled cash accounts both of which are mechanisms for control and reduction of capital investments in building programs.

A third point in the cost containment effort is to ask all medical staffs to re-affirm their commitment to voluntary utilization review programs and further tighten the programs. Some hospital systems operate under an open staff concept where a physician from one member hospital is automatically extended privileges to work in other member hospitals. In addition, the existence of joint or cooperative medical staffs in systems allows for consolidation of patient care information toward systemwide quality assurance programs. This larger data base affords systems the opportunity to set standards which are based on centralized information from multiple facilities. The establishment of performance standards by systemwide bases theoretically results in higher quality of care and a greater commitment on the part of physicians to the delivery of the higher standard patient care. The consolidation of committee responsibility, data gathering and analysis contributes to further cost avoidance on a system basis.

A two percent improvement in hospital productivity per year is another goal of the voluntary effort. Many hospital systems have implemented systemwide productivity standards which relate staffing to degree and volume of patient activities.

These are but a few of many examples where multihospital systems can contribute a great deal more to the effectiveness of legislation or regulation than the single freestanding institution.

The Application of Existing and Proposed Laws and Regulations to the Development of Multihospital Systems

This conference has already noted the several positive thrusts towards further development and incentives for development of multihospital systems. Specifically, we have noted that Secretary Califano recently acknowledged that "Current Medicare reimbursement provides little incentive for nonprofit providers to established shared services since Medicare reimbursement is reduced dollar for dollar as a result of any savings made."

We concur with Mr. Califano's statement except that it does not go far enough. In some cases, existing regulation and proposed regulation serve to actively discourage the formation and operation of multihospital systems. This next section of the presentation is intended to clarify some of the areas in which the application of existing and proposed laws and regulation are in conflict with the policy goal of encouraging the development of multihospital systems. We recognize that much of the existing law and regulations were drawn prior to the development of multihospital systems. However, if the government wishes to encourage the development of these systems as part of its cost containment strategy, existing disincentives will have to be removed and positive incentives will have to be created to foster the growth of multihospital systems. Rather than attempt an exhaustive listing and detailing of all problem areas related to multihospital system development, let me use four areas which currently have a negative impact upon multihospital system development:

- The impact of piecemeal regulation
- Restrictions on capital accumulation and use
- Cost containment disincentives
- Restrictions on corporate form and scope of activities

Impact of Piecemeal Regulation

Existing and proposed health industry regulation is oriented toward the individual provider. With a possible exception of the Rostenkowski/Rogers proposals, regulators have demonstrated an unwillingness to review an entire hospital system rather than its component providers. The Rostenkowski/Rogers proposals provide that hospitals may be consolidated, provided they are within the same HEW region. This option, although a first step in the right direction, again ignores the way in which a multihospital system really operates by placing arbitrary geographical limitations on the option.

The following examples will illustrate further the impact of piecemeal regulation:

- Allowability of lay equivalent salaries. . . . The Medicare program is challenging allowability of lay equivalent salary reimbursement in the mother house or corporate offices of Catholic owned multihospital systems. This challenge is based upon the Medicare program's interpretation of original regulation as defining reimbursement only for Sisters located at providers and not for Sisters located outside the hospitals. This appears to be a very narrow arbitrary challenge with no apparent intent or desire to review benefits provided on a systemwide basis.

- Medicare home office cost report proposal. . . . In its recent proposal with respect to home office cost reports, the Medicare program has ignored obvious differences between large and small hospital systems, proprietary versus not-for-profit hospital systems, and urban based systems versus rural based systems in trying to require onerous reporting of data which, in many cases, is not germane to specific types of systems.

- Balance sheet reporting requirements. . . . The program requires that individual hospital balance sheets be filed by members of nonprofit multihospital systems. Although many systems have consolidated their assets into a single organization and, therefore, have only a single balance sheet and, therefore, balance sheets are not used for individual hospitals in the system and have no real meaning, the Medicare program has refused to review the multihospital system as a whole and has continued to look at individual hospitals.

- Appeal mechanisms. . . . Presently, there is no mechanism whereby a multihospital corporation can appeal a Medicare issue on behalf of all of it providers. It must select a single provider and use it as a vehicle to appeal the issue, even though that issue has equal applicability to all of the system's units.

- Reimbursement limitations. . . . Presently, the lower of cost or charges limitation and routine services limitation are applied on a facility by facility basis, instead of a systemwide basis. Such limitations could more equitably apply for an entire system without any loss of overall regulatory control.

These issues are merely illustrations of a common approach in which the Medicare program examines bits and pieces of multihospital systems operations, rather than attempting to look at the system as an entity. There is no apparent attempt to look at the benefits of a multihospital system as they relate to the operation of individual providers. Certain costs must be incurred in multihospital system central offices to lower costs in the entire system, and it is from this overall benefit evaluation prospective that reimbursement should be examined rather than from a narrow, piecemeal prospective.

Restrictions on Capital Accumulation and Use

If any organization is to continue to exist, it must be able to accumulate from operations some portion of the capital required to finance replacements and needed growth. Nonprofit hospital systems are prohibited from accumulating capital in excess of depreciation amounts from the Medicare portion of their operations. Furthermore, they are regulated as to how they use capital accumulated from any and all sources. These factors can be explained in more depth through the following comments:

- Capital planning. . . . The Medicare program is very punitive with regard to sound financial planning for capital accumulation. Specifically, the funded depreciation regulations have forced providers to deplete cash reserves before allowing reimbursement of interest expense on borrowed funds. One of the major benefits of a multihospital system is its ability to accumulate capital on a system-wide basis and then to allocate that capital for use in various projects at times which must be determined based on sound capital and financial planning. Current regulations preclude such planning and thus hamper the possibility and effectiveness of the operations of a multihospital system.
- Capital fund accumulation. . . . The Medicare and Medicaid programs currently pay for services provided to Medicare and Medicaid patients based upon cost reimbursement. This allows for no excess of revenue over expenses to be accumulated on the Medicare/Medicaid services provided. This nonallowance of some amount of revenues over expenses is extremely detrimental to the future financial viability of individual hospitals and multihospital systems. The only dollars which these programs allow to be utilized for future capital needs become dollars generated through funding of historical cost depreciation. Such dollars are obviously insufficient to meet capital replacement and expansion needs for several reasons. First, inflation, both as it applies to the general economy and, more specifically, as it applies to the health care industry,

makes replacement costs much higher than historical costs. Second, with ever increasing sophistication in technology, replacement costs are substantially increased. Third, dollars to be utilized for necessary planning agency approved expansion do not become available under this system. Therefore, the nonallowance of some amount of revenues over expenses and the nonallowance of current value depreciation as opposed to historical cost depreciation effectively restrict accumulation of capital funds to a level threatening the viability of multihospital systems.

By disallowing the accumulation of cash reserves to meet the above needs over and above funded depreciation, Medicare and Medicaid programs force other patients to pay disproportionately for their services in order to accumulate necessary capital funds. Recent studies conducted by several multihospital systems show that this disproportionate payment by private patients amounts to at least $15 per patient per day and in some instances over $50 per patient per day to make up for the Medicare/Medicaid difference. This is obviously inequitable as Medicare/Medicaid patients will also be using the facility in the future. In extreme cases where Medicare/Medicaid utilization is very high, this forced nonaccumulation of necessary cash reserves will lead to eventual hospital closure.

Cost Containment Disincentives

One of the major disincentives for the formation and growth of nonprofit multihospital systems is the opportunity to contain or reduce costs. The reduction in Medicare reimbursement matching the reduction in cost provides an overall disincentive to multihospital arrangements. But, in addition to this overall disincentive, there are several specific disincentives built into existing regulations. For example:

- Medicare management contract proposed regulations. . . . In its recent proposal with respect to the reimbursability of management contract fees, it appears that the Medicare program has gone out of its way to make the management contract arrangement difficult rather than providing any incentives for this type of multihospital system arrangement.
- Medicare reimbursement principles on self-insurance. . . . By limiting or denying reimbursement of expenses under self-insurance plans, the program has effectively discouraged the development of such plans which have great potential for cost savings. This approach has had a particular impact on multihospital systems,

because they have been the leaders in developing such plans and are more likely to have a large insured population for risk spreading.

Restrictions on Corporate Form and Scope of Activities

Nonprofit multihospital systems presently operate in a confusing and complex legal environment. Two major areas of legal concern are antitrust law and the income tax code.

- Antitrust concerns. . . . There is a general concern among multihospital system managers that any joint action by a group of hospitals that would impact hospital charges or costs in a geographical area could be construed as anticompetitive behavior. This concern stems from proposals emanating from governmental agencies such as the Justice Department and the Federal Trade Commission and have caused multihospital systems to be limited in expanding their activities into new geographical areas or into new shared service activities.

- Internal Revenue concerns. . . . If a nonprofit multihospital system enters into certain types of contracts which would reduce overall hospital costs, it could jeopardize its nonprofit status. Specifically, contracts or employment arrangements which reward individuals for performance against established monetary objectives may be construed to be providing inurement to the benefit of an individual from the operation of the organization. Such an arrangement, although very common as a compensation practice, and although having potential cost containment and efficiency benefits, could cause the organization to lose it tax exempt status.

Unrelated business income is another Internal Revenue concern to multihospital systems. Services provided to a nonowned or controlled facility may give rise to unrelated business income and, therefore, a tax liability. This is true even if the nonowned facility is also a nonprofit organization.

The Internal Revenue has taken the position that income relating to services shared by one nonprofit hospital organization with another nonowned, nonprofit hospital is unrelated business income and is taxable to the first hospital. This is true even though both hospitals are nonprofit and the sharing results in reduced overall costs. Although this position has been successfully challenged in the courts and has been overturned in specific instances, such as the United Hospital laundry case, substantial uncertainty remains as to whether or not shared services to nonowned facilities give rise to unrelated business income and a tax liability. Thus, there is a potential penalty assessed for attempting to share services and reduce costs.

General Issues of Legislation and Regulation in the Areas of Health Finance, Health Planning, and Quality of Care

There are many general issues relating to legislation and regulation in the other topic areas to be discussed in this conference. We have discussed some of the areas in health finance, so let's briefly look at general issues in the other two areas, health planning and quality of care.

While at least 3 of the 10 National Priorities stated in Section 1502 of Public Law 93-641 relate to the further developments of multi-institutional arrangements, there has been little done to date which would clarify how the health planning process is designed to contribute to this development.

Health Systems Agencies should have access to knowledge and technical expertise to encourage the development of shared services or effectively contribute to the further development of integrated hospital systems.

Duplicative review costs may currently be incurred where multiple hospitals involved in one project must apply to multiple HSAs for approval, thereby negating some of the savings which can accrue due to centralized planning on a systemwide basis.

Further research is required to more fully document the advantages and potential disadvantages of shared services in multihospital systems. This should be one of the priorities of the regional centers with respect to health planning. In the area of quality of care, there are also several general issues. The balancing of cost consideration and quality of care are difficult issues for the provider alone. Other sectors such as government and the planning process must also be involved in this delicate balancing act.

Flexibility in the development of quality assurance programs is essential. No one structure for a quality assurance program is correct for all health facilities, particularly for multihospital systems which have entirely different operating mechanisms.

Reimbursement for joint activities in a hospital system and continued access to debt financing will continue to have major impact upon the quality of care in a hospital system.

A Summary of Projections or Suggestions for the Future

This presentation has attempted to outline some of the strengths and weaknesses of multihospital systems and how they impact or can impact upon the health legislation and regulatory process. There are several additional suggestions that might be made for future consideration.

- Multihospital systems would like to encourage the Congress, its staff, and the federal agencies to work with The Center for Multihospital Systems and Shared Service Organizations to remove those disincentives which operate to discourage systems development. Also, those disincentives which work to decrease the operating advantages of a multihospital system should be carefully studied and improvements made where possible.
- Multihospital systems and legislators/regulators should jointly develop positive incentives to foster the appropriate growth of systems. We are encouraged and pleased with the beginning steps toward the creation of positive incentives evidenced recently. These include: Secretary Califano's statement on the proposed change in Medicare reimbursement on shared services; the Rostenkowski/Rogers proposals on the treatment of multihospital systems contained within HR 6575; and Assistant Secretary Derzon's comments on encouraging the development of multihospital systems and other similar encouragements.
- We would like to encourage federal agencies and Congress to utilize the interest and strengths of the multihospital system's approach in developing the necessary health legislation initiatives and the appropriate regulation to implement that legislation. I can assure you the interest of the systems in working with you in this effort is high and can be sustained.
- Utilize the hospital systems to test the impact of regulations in such areas as cost benefit analysis with a particular set of regulations. Again there are many willing and able systems available to you for this effort.
- Within the federal agencies and the Congress, work to remove the uncertainty and the contradiction in health regulations which confuse or thwart the effect of systems benefits.
- Assist hospitals and hospital systems through legislative initiatives to attack the real causes of hospital cost increase. Such areas as unlimited health care demands, inappropriate supply and distribution of health facilities, and costs imposed upon the health system from other sectors of the economy are important areas worth study. This type of legislative initiative, as opposed to the papering over of the symptoms with more costly and duplicative regulations, is an effort that has great potential yield in results.

In conclusion, it is important to leave you with the attitude that I'm sure prevails among managers of multihospital systems with regard to health legislation and health regulation. What we are seeking is a partnership, not a pitched battle.

REFERENCES

1. Phillips, Donald F. and Kessler, Marian S. "Criticism of the Medicare Validation Survey." *Hospitals, J.A.H.A.* 49:61-66, September 1, 1975.